SAFE ALTERNATIVES in CHILDBIRTH

Cover Photo Caption.

First Love

28 minutes into life, searching eyes,
    Asking "Who?"
Father's firm hands, vibrant velvet bodylet.
    We accept.
I, you; you, me. Wordless we recognize.

D. Stewart

National
Association of
Parents & Professionals for
Safe
Alternatives in
Childbirth

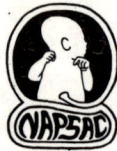

SAFE ALTERNATIVES IN CHILDBIRTH

edited by

David Stewart, PhD
& Lee Stewart, CCE

CONTRIBUTING AUTHORS

George J. Annas, JD, MPH
James D. Brew, MD, FACOG
Hart Collins
Neil Collins, JD
Ludovic J. DeVocht, MD, ACOG
Mayer Eisenstein, MD, ACHO
Janet Epstein, RN, CNM
Frederic Ettner, MD, ACHO
Doris Haire, DMS
Cedar Koons
Stephen Koons

Betty Hosford, RN, CNM
Martha Longbrake, RN
William Longbrake, DBA
Ruth Watson Lubic, RN, CNM
Marion F. McCartney, RN, CNM
Lewis E. Mehl, MD, ACHO
Robert Mendelsohn, MD, ACHO
Nancy Mills, Lay Midwife
Lee Stewart, BS, CCE
David Stewart, CCE, PHD
Marian Tompson, LLLI

Based On The

FIRST AMERICAN NAPSAC CONFERENCE
May 15, 1976, Arlington, Virginia

Overlooking the Nation's Capital, Washington, D.C.

Indexed By
Jamy Braun, RN

Published By

NAPSAC, INC.
CHAPEL HILL, NC

First Edition, June 1976, 2,000 copies
Second Edition, February 1977, 5,000 copies
Third Edition, January 1978, 5,000 copies

Library of Congress Number: 76-19336
ISBN 0-917314-06-9

Available from: NAPSAC   After June 1, 1978, Order From
                  P.O. Box 1307   NAPSAC
                  Chapel Hill, NC 27514   P.O. Box 267
                  (Until June 1, 1978)   Marble Hill, MO 63764

Price: $5.00   (plus 50¢ shipping & handling if ordered direct
                  from publisher)

*All proceeds from this book go toward the accomplishment of the goals
of NAPSAC (see p. 184), a non-profit, tax exempt service corporation.
None of the 22 authors receive royalties. All generously contributed
their time and work to produce this anthology. Among other things,
the book is a monument to their dedication to the betterment of our
society through more humane maternity care.*

Printed in the U.S.A.
by the CAROLINA COPY CENTER, Chapel Hill, NC

*   CONTRIBUTIONS TO NAPSAC ARE TAX DEDUCTIBLE

TABLE OF CONTENTS

FORWARD

This book is the result of a National Conference entitled "Safe Alternatives in Childbirth " held May 15, 1976, in Arlington, Virginia, adjacent to the Pentagon and overlooking the United States Capital, Washington, DC. It was the First American Conference to be sponsored by NAPSAC - The National Association of Parents & Professionals for Safe Alternatives in Childbirth.

The conference was attended by over 500 persons from 28 States, Canada, and Australia. Represented there were nurses, lay midwives, nurse midwives, obstetricians, pediatricians, family practitioners, chiropractors, osteopaths, lawyers, authors, news writers, La Leche League leaders, childbirth educators, public health officials, social workers, psychologists, fathers, and mothers.

The content of this book is based upon a transcript of the conference as well as additional written materials submitted by the various conference participants. Some of the articles published here consist entirely of an edited tape transcript, others entirely of written materials submitted by the author(s), and others are based on both, submitted written material and transcribed spoken word, combined into a single article by the editors. The presentations of David Stewart, Frederic Ettner, Lewis Mehl, Hart & Neil Collins, and Martha & William Longbrake are based entirely on written materials by the respective authors. The presentations of Lee Stewart, Doris Haire, Mayer Eisenstein, Nancy Mills, and Cedar & Stephen Koons are based entirely on the transcribed tapes of their talks at the conference. The presentations of Betty Hosford, Ruth Lubic, Robert Mendelsohn, Janet Epstein, et al., Marian Tompson, and George Annas are based upon a combination of written materials and transcribed spoken words. In the case of George Annas, the written material used was copyrighted but used here with permission (see note on p. 161).

In editing the transcribed tapes for this publication, extraneous comments appropriately made at the conference were deleted and minor revisions of grammar and syntax were made to effect the metamorphosis from the spoken format into the written. Throughout the book selected quotes are displayed in bold type. In these instances, the quotes are either extracted verbatum or paraphrased from the article in which the quote appears except in some instances where quotes made by the author verbally are only displayed in the bold format without repetition in the finer text. Unless otherwise noted, all such quotes are attributable to the author(s) in whose article they appear.

This book contains a variety of thoughts, some even contradictory, and is not intended to be a completely coherent work with a consistent theme. The opinions stated here are those of the various authors and are not necessarily those of NAPSAC. For questions on any of the content found here, please write directly to the author concerned. A complete list of addresses is given on page 182.

Considerable effort has been expended to make this book as useable as possible at as reasonable a cost as feasible and in as short a time following the Conference as could be managed. In all, it only took 6 weeks from the day of the Conference to obtain the first printing from the press. Because of the speed with which this was accomplished and because of the reliance upon taped, verbal presentations, there may be mis-spelled names and/or other errors. We plan to have future printings so if you find errors, we would appreciate your passing the information along to us so that we can correct them for subsequent editions.

Although not intended to be, in any sense, a comprehensive account of "Alternatives in Childbirth," we feel that the book does offer a new breadth of viewpoints on certain childbirth options that is presently not available in print. Along with the inspirational and philosophical articles, there are also those of facts and numbers, as well as details and statistics of working alternative programs to the hospital regime. For example, contained in these pages are the working details of a Childbearing Center in New York City; a well-worked-out homebirth program led by nurse midwives in Washington, DC; an urban physicians' home obstetric service in Chicago; the means and practices of lay midwives in California; as well as information on several physician-nurse family practice groups that offer choices of care to their mothers--from hospital to home.

For physicians, nurses, midwives, interns, residents, or medical students seeking information and support in the field of home obstetrics, there is a section of the book (p. 183) describing the American College of Home Obstetrics.

Until communities offer *good alternatives* in maternity services, parents have no real "freedom of choice." Other volumes will be added to this one as NAPSAC has major conferences in the future. Until then, we offer this, our first, with the hope that you will find it helpful in obtaining the maternity programs you need for your area--be it more family-centered hospitals, a childbearing center, or a safe homebirth program--so that you may obtain the kind of childbirth you desire and deserve for you, your children, your family, and your community.

The Editors
David & Lee Stewart
Hillsborough, NC
June 1976

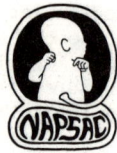

ACKNOWLEDGEMENTS

We wish to express our appreciation to the many persons who offered helpful suggestions for the second edition.

In particular, we appreciate the corrections written to us by EVA REICH, MD, *and which have been incorporated into this edition.*

And we especially appreciate the work of Ms. DIONY YOUNG, *medical editor and journalist, who generously contributed her time and expertise to make corrections and suggestions for the book. Meticulously proofreading every paragraph and table for correct grammer, spelling, usage, and punctuation--she submitted over 500 corrections and suggestions which have been incorporated into this present edition. Of particular importance was her checking of all medical terms for spelling and usage. The improvements of this second edition over the first are, thus, to a large extent, due to the dedicated, careful work of* Ms. Young. *Thank you,* Diony.

David & Lee Stewart, Editors
Hillsborough, NC
January 1977

Opening Address

HOMEBIRTHS - A MODERN TREND - IS IT PROGRESS?

David Stewart, PhD, CCE*

Hospitals have never been proven to be the safest place for most mothers to give birth to their babies. In fact, available evidence suggests that quite the contrary may be true. As you will see by the presentations here, there is strong evidence to suggest that a maternity program that would result in the best medical, psychological, and sociological outcome would be one that offered parents choices of alternatives. These choices would include:

(1) Good hospitals, for those few who truly need or desire them, with true family centered policies (not just token programs as many now have) and

(2) Childbearing centers and good, well-thought-out homebirth programs for the majority.

It is not our purpose, at this time, to prove that homebirths are as safe as hospital births because presently there are not sufficient data to prove one way or the other. But neither are there sufficient data to prove that hospitals are as safe as is popularly believed. No study has ever been made demonstrating that routine hospitalization of birthing mothers results in statistically improved medical outcomes when compared to a comprehensive consumer-oriented maternity program offering alternatives. And no data will become available for such a comparative study until *after* well-planned maternity centers and carefully handled homebirth programs have been allowed to operate freely for a period of years. Until then the pros and cons are only theoretical and theory can never be conclusive either way. After all, who waited for hospitals to conclusively prove themselves *before* implementing massive institutional maternity programs?

If you study the process whereby new medical ideas become "proven practice" you will observe that there are two distinct phases: *First*, the new idea is tested as best it can by application of reason to available facts and, where appropriate, it is tested by laboratory experiments ending with a limited number of trials on human subjects. But this first stage, no matter how thorough, can never be conclusive. It can only weed out the ideas that are clearly not good for gross reasons. At some stage, when a new idea fails to be rejected from clear theoretical or laboratory evidence, it must be tried upon human

---

* DAVID STEWART *is Director of the MacCarthy Geophysics Laboratory, University of North Carolina; U.S. Southern Regional Director, International Childbirth Education Association; U.S. Southeastern Area Coordinator, American Academy of Husband-Coached Childbirth; Author (with his wife's assistance) of the pamphlet, "Father To Father On Breastfeeding," published by La Leche League International; Father of five children--all by medically unattended homebirths; Cofounder and Executive Director, NAPSAC, and Chairman of the First American NAPSAC Conference.*

HOMEBIRTH TREND   -2-

subjects in large numbers under clinical conditions.   This is the
Second stage of research. Unfortunately, it is not always recognized
as a "stage of research" since, at this point, the public is often led
to believe that the procedure has been "proven." But no medical practice can be considered proven more beneficial than harmful until *after*
years of application by hundreds of doctors on thousands of patients.

NO STUDY HAS EVER BEEN MADE DEMONSTRATING THAT ROUTINE
HOSPITALIZATION OF BIRTHING MOTHERS RESULTS IN STATISTI-
CALLY IMPROVED MEDICAL OUTCOMES WHEN COMPARED TO A COMPREHENSIVE
CONSUMER-ORIENTED MATERNITY PROGRAM OFFERING ALTERNATIVES.

Innumerable examples of this two-step testing process exist in
medical history. In recent times, diuretics prescribed in pregnancy
were so tested for many years only to be found, after millions had
been affected, that such drugs can do irreparable damage to the fetus.
Similarly with diethylstilbestrol (DES)--a drug thought relatively
harmless and with certain benefits to mothers about to miscarry, when
it was discovered after decades of use that DES was responsible for
certain cancers. Today we are in the midst of several new research
experiments upon mothers and babies. As examples, I cite the routine
use of fetal monitors and the increased application of C-sections.
Will fetal monitors and higher C-section rates eventually prove more
beneficial than harmful when compared to alternatives?   Who knows?
Only after many years and countless mothers and babies so tested will
the data really be available for doctors to know for sure.

Therefore, there is nothing unusual in proposing that homebirth
programs and maternity centers be tried with vigor and made available
to large masses of the people where desired. They have certainly passed
the *first* stage of medical research. Their validity as safe alternatives
is at least as well established as the current push to regionalize perinatal services or the wide use of fetal monitors, increased C-section
rates, frequent artificial rupture of membranes, and a host of other
widely used obstetrical practices. Hence, there can be *no* grounds for
objection to these alternatives *based on fact* since the facts are not
complete, and never will be until *after* some years of their actual application. We are merely proposing that the same standard of scientific
validation the medical establishment routinely applies to itself be also
applied to *Alternatives in Childbirth*.

WHAT MOTHERS' FEELINGS HAVE BEEN TELLING US FOR CENTURIES
SHOULD BE ASSUMED TO BE CORRECT UNTIL PROVEN OTHERWISE.

Another obstacle to beneficial change in maternity practice is
the common attitude, on the part of many of the public and the medical
community alike, which assumes that physicians' feelings and established
hospital traditions should be presumed to be correct until proven otherwise. I propose that we should adopt the attitude that what mothers'
feelings have been telling us for centuries should be assumed to be
correct until proven otherwise. The time has come for hospitals to
defend, or desist doing, what they have been doing for decades without
scientific basis.

"Homebirths - A Modern Trend - Is It Progress?" The title of my presentation poses two questions: (1) Is it really a trend? and (2) Is it progress? My wife, Lee, and I have been watching the growth of homebirth interest in the United States for many years--ever since the pregnancy of our first child born at home 13 years ago tomorrow (May 16, 1963). We have had five children at home all told--the last only three months ago (February 8, 1976). During the past 13 years we have communicated with hundreds of couples about homebirths. They write, visit, and call in ever increasing numbers every year. During the past three years a number of new nation-wide organizations have been founded to support homebirth programs--many of which are represented here at this conference today. Believe me--it is no fad. Homebirth is a real trend and it is going to continue at an increasing rate whether physicians, nurses, nurse midwives, professional childbirth educators, and public health officials want to participate in it or not.

> HOMEBIRTH IS A REAL TREND, NOT A FAD, AND IT IS GOING TO CONTINUE AT AN INCREASING RATE WHETHER HEALTH PROFESSIONALS WANT TO PARTICIPATE IN IT OR NOT.

Is it progress? Definitely yes. Why? Because it is the manifestation of greater awareness and concern on the part of today's parents. In our experience, it is usually the parents who are the most informed and who care the most for the safety of their baby who choose a homebirth. Those parents who are least informed usually relinquish themselves to doctors and hospitals without question, thus abdicating their responsibility and, unknown to them, also giving up their divine birthright to one of life's most potentially uplifting experiences.

> IT IS USUALLY THE PARENTS WHO ARE THE MOST INFORMED AND WHO CARE THE MOST FOR THE SAFETY OF THEIR BABY WHO CHOOSE A HOMEBIRTH. THOSE WHO ARE LEAST INFORMED USUALLY RELINQUISH THEMSELVES TO DOCTORS AND HOSPITALS WITHOUT QUESTION.

Victor Hugo once said, "There is no idea so powerful as one whose time has come." The time has come to implement *Alternatives in Childbirth*. The very fact that this conference is happening now proves it. In fact, so many wanted to come we almost had to turn people away. We only planned for 300 and there are well over 500 here from 28 states and Canada. Only by some last minute rearrangements were we able to accommodate such an enthusiastic turnout.

Today may well prove to be a historic one in the progress of maternity practice. It is my privilege and pleasure to welcome you to be a part of it. Thank you.

Why Is There A Need For Alternatives in Childbirth?

Lee Stewart, BS, CCE*

I was born on a farm near Lutesville, Missouri, a small town of 600 population then and 600 population now. It was Christmas morning in 1937. My brother, who was three years old, woke up that morning, passed up all the presents that Santa had brought, and went straight in to see his newly arrived baby sister--me. There I was, brand new, barely dry, and in bed with my mother--available for my brother to come in and see and touch and welcome. My father was there to cook his usual eggs and pork and beans. That's one thing that Daddy could cook and I remember we had it every time Mom gave birth.

Compare this scene to another hypothetical one with which most of you are probably more familiar. The three year old child would wake up Christmas morning and his mother would be gone. She would be in a hospital with a new baby, something he's not sure he understands. A baby that he cannot see or touch. Neither can he see his mother. In this scene, neither would the three year old be interested in his Christmas presents, but not because of his joy and interest in the new baby, but because of his confusion and panic that his mother is missing. And the father, also separated, has to cope with this uncopeable situation.

My remembrance of birth is positive. Mom had four more children in that old farm house. My remembrance of birth was to wake up and find a baby in bed with my mother, and Daddy taking care of Mom. It was always very exciting. No one in our family knew what it was like to experience jealous feelings for a new baby. I didn't realize such jealousy existed until I was in college and people talked about "sibling rivalry." My mother didn't talk of birth at all except when asked and then to say that childbirth is very painful, that women would not have babies were it not for maternal amnesia. But it was the attitude of birth that stuck with me. The positive attitude of birth in the home surroundings, early and close, father, mother, infant, sibling contact. Every baby welcomed and loved.

Women in those days gave birth in the proper surroundings for positive attitudes but were untrained to handle the process of birth. Women today are trained, but much of that training is how to cope with the unfamiliar surroundings of the hospital. Have you childbirth educators ever stopped to think how much time is spent in class teaching women and couples to cope with hospitals instead of merely teaching about the birth process?

---

* LEE STEWART is U.S. Southern Regional Director, International Childbirth Education Association; U.S. Southeastern Area Coordinator, American Academy of Husband-Coached Childbirth; La Leche League Leader, and, although not listed as a coauthor on the LLLI pamphlet #128 for fathers, she edited it, wrote several parts of it, and provided the essential education and inspiration to her husband, Dave, who could not have otherwise written it; Mother of five children--all medically unattended homebirths; Cofounder and President of NAPSAC.

HAVE YOU CHILDBIRTH EDUCATORS EVER STOPPED TO THINK HOW MUCH CLASS TIME IS SPENT TEACHING COUPLES TO COPE WITH HOSPITALS INSTEAD OF MERELY TEACHING ABOUT THE BIRTH PROCESS?

Tomorrow is the 13th birthday of our oldest son.   Thirteen years ago we chose an unattended homebirth in preference to traditional hospital birth. When we approached a doctor for prenatal care we found that the doctor knew nothing of natural childbirth. Women were routinely anesthetized. Dave wanted to be there at the birth. We were informed that this was impossible. "The delivery room was too small." They would not even talk about the baby being able to be with me upon birth. When we found that our strong desires and feelings could not be met, even talked about, we dropped the bomb with our next question: "Well, what do you think about having the baby at home?" The doctor walked out of the room and we were dismissed. As we left his office we were requested to pay his usual $5.

We decided that it was impossible to buck the established routine of a hospital. We tried to find a doctor who would attend our birth at home but none would even think of coming. We knew there were *possible* risks of having our baby at home unattended by a doctor, but we also knew the risks of a hospital birth and many of these were not just possibilities, but *certainties*. Thirteen years ago in Warrensburg, Missouri, there was the *real risk* of routine anesthesia which could not be avoided in that hospital. There were the *certain risks* of routine separation of mother, father, and baby--the psychological risks of this separation are only recently coming into view through studies. If we would have had to wait for scientific studies on how we got pregnant and how a baby develops inside before we did it, the human race would be extinct. I am glad we didn't wait for these studies of early and close infant contact to follow what we felt to be right.

It has been interesting for us to note that women and couples are faced with the same choices today despite our progress in childbirth and childbirth education. Women still have to fight to have natural childbirth. Fathers still have to fight to be with their wife during labor and birth. Women *still* have to fight to have their baby with them--*of all things!* We have been told that what we encountered over 13 years ago that made us choose a homebirth isn't a problem these days. But I talk to women every day who are still encountering these attitudes. The choice, in most places, is still between a compromised hospital birth or an unattended homebirth sometimes even without prenatal care because of the refusal of some physicians.

IF WE WOULD HAVE HAD TO WAIT FOR SCIENTIFIC STUDIES ON HOW WE GOT PREGNANT AND HOW A BABY DEVELOPS INSIDE BEFORE WE DID IT, THE HUMAN RACE WOULD BE EXTINCT.

After our first baby was born, we have had positive help and support as far as prenatal care and all of our questions have been answered by friendly and helpful doctors and nurses. Our criteria for our first birth could now be met in the hospital in our area. But now we have something else we think is very important--*sibling* participation. Jonathan, our oldest son, has been present and involved in the births of his sister and three brothers. Lora Lee has seen three births, Keith--two, and Ben--one. Their response to birth is positive and they wouldn't miss it.

Just to give you an idea of a child's reaction to birth, three year old Lora Lee, as she saw Keith tumble out before her eyes, said, "Daddy, what is that?" We never could convince her that, indeed, there was a baby growing inside of Mommy. She would look at me and say, "Sure, I have a baby in my belly too." She later said she thought Keith was a turtle. When Ben was born, Keith, who was two at the time, exclaimed, "Look Mom. He's naked!"

If a child is allowed to be involved in the birth of his brother or sister and *actually sees the baby emerge* from the mother, we feel that the child will realize that the baby is physically a part of the mother and will have no trouble accepting the baby just as he has already accepted his mother.

WHEN BEN WAS BORN, OUR TWO YEAR OLD, KEITH, EXCLAIMED, "LOOK, MOM. HE'S NAKED!"

We have had five unattended homebirths because there have been no homebirth programs where we have lived, nor has there been a doctor nor a midwife who would attend our births. Nor could the hospital meet what we felt was vitally important for the birth and health of our children. We are having our babies now. We can't wait 20 years until studies point the way for more humane childbirth practices.

WE ARE HAVING OUR BABIES NOW. WE CAN'T WAIT 20 YEARS UNTIL STUDIES POINT THE WAY TO MORE HUMANE CHILDBIRTH PRACTICES.

WHY IS THERE A NEED FOR ALTERNATIVES?   First, we question that hospitals are in the best interest and optimum safety of all mothers and families giving birth. The hospital is an unfamiliar situation and an unfamiliar place. This, in itself, can contribute to longer labors and problems in birth. Many women are more afraid of the unfamiliar hospital surroundings than they are of the birth process itself. In the hospital there are strangers managing things for you. Most women have not had continuity of care with one doctor or midwife. In clinic situations, in our area at least, a woman may never have even met the resident who handles her labor and delivers her baby. And in many private practice situations, there is little difference from the discontinuous care of the clinics. Very few obstetricians seem to realize how important it is for us to know and to have confidence in the person who helps us manage labor and catches our baby.

The hospital is a place of germs and disease. One of the prime objections I have heard against homebirth is that of unsanitary conditions in the home. But, as a matter of fact, most infections of mother and baby are caused by the hospital environment itself.

Another big argument against homebirth is that the hospital is equipped to handle emergencies. The home is not. The coin is always two-sided. *Because* the hospital is equipped to handle emergencies, *more risks are taken*. Therefore, the hospital poses risks that are unique and unheard-of at home. Let me give some examples.

MANY WOMEN ARE MORE AFRAID OF THE UNFAMILIAR HOSPITAL SURROUNDINGS THAN THEY ARE OF THE BIRTH PROCESS ITSELF.

Prenatal care is not approached from as preventive an angle as it could because if an emergency happens in a hospital, they feel that they can take care of it. Just think how different prenatal care would have to be for a good homebirth program to work--how improved prenatal care would be.

More medication is used with less discrimination in hospitals because if there is a problem due to the medication, the hospital has the equipment and staff to handle an emergency--*or so they think*. Of necessity natural childbirth would have to be practiced in a safe home birth program. If a woman has need of medication, she should be in the hospital. But I might point out that Dr. Grantly Dick-Read trained well over 90% of the women to go through labor and birth without medication. And so does Dr. Robert Bradley--presently practicing.

More obstetrical intervention takes place in the hospital environment *because* they feel they are equipped to handle it if something goes wrong. Would membranes be ruptured routinely in homebirth? Would episiotomies be performed so routinely or haphazardly? There are these things, and many others, done routinely in the hospital with very little thought that they wouldn't dare do, or at least I hope they wouldn't dare do, in a homebirth because the hospital is equipped to handle emergencies.

BECAUSE THE HOSPITAL IS EQUIPPED TO HANDLE EMERGENCIES, MORE RISKS ARE TAKEN. THEREFORE, THE HOSPITAL POSES RISKS THAT ARE UNIQUE AND UNHEARD-OF AT HOME.

WHY IS THERE A NEED FOR ALTERNATIVES? The cost of hospital birth has reached phenomenal heights. Cost is something that no one wants to talk about. Somehow we're supposed to be beyond that. But like it or not, cost is something that is woven throughout our whole system. The cost of a normal birth in our area is about $1,000. In other areas it can be more than double this amount. It is interesting to note that the Maternity Center Association in New York City and the Maternity Center Associates in Washington, DC, can provide more personal and complete care for about half the hospital costs in our area.

> THERE ARE NO SAFE HOMEBIRTHS WITHOUT GOOD HOSPITALS NEARBY, BUT WE FEEL THAT EVERYONE SHOULD NOT HAVE TO CONFORM TO BIRTH IN THE HOSPITAL. THERE SHOULD BE SAFE SENSIBLE CHOICES.

Third, to offer alternatives in childbirth fits the needs of a broader spectrum of people. I don't want you to get the wrong idea from this presentation. We in NAPSAC are not trying to do away with hospitals. There are no safe homebirths without good hospitals nearby, but we feel that everyone should not have to conform to birth in the hospital. Birth is a very personal thing. We think there should be safe, sensible choices. While you need good hospitals to back up homebirth programs, hospitals also need good homebirth programs to give them a base of normality by which to measure and stimulate more truly family centered care. Ideally, we would like to see family centered care in hospitals, childbearing centers, and good homebirth programs working hand in hand for the benefit of parents and babies. There are qualified professionals interested in providing these alternatives and there are parents interested in taking advantage of such programs.

> ANYTIME THERE IS MONOPOLY OF POWER, THERE IS SMALL INCENTIVE TO MAKE CHANGES TO FIT PEOPLE'S NEEDS. BUT IF ALTERNATIVES ARE PROVIDED, PEOPLE MAY CHOOSE AND THIS WOULD ENCOURAGE POSITIVE IMPROVEMENTS IN ALL ALTERNATIVES.

Fourth, competition causes improvements. This is another aspect that some people do not like to talk about, especially those currently in power. Anytime there is a monopoly of power, there is small incentive to make changes to fit people's needs. But if alternatives are provided, people may choose and this would encourage positive improvements in all alternatives.

Fifth, routine hospital birth has caused doctors and obstetricians to see birth in a clinical, pathological manner instead of as a natural function. Most doctors who handle birth these days have never seen a natural childbirth. Most are surprised to learn of a woman who has given birth without an episiotomy and without perineal or vaginal laceration. A popular comment to that is "You were lucky!" The concept of routine IVs, pushing the baby out in the supine position with your feet in stirrups, and many other non-natural practices are seen by hospital-trained doctors as normal. How many doctors graduating from medical school have seen a true natural childbirth--even though they may work with prepared couples? How many doctors, even though they have practiced for years, have seen the beautiful outcome for mother and baby of a true natural birth?

> THE OUTCOME OF BIRTH IS ONLY IN THE HANDS OF THE OBSTETRICIAN AND THE HOSPITAL STAFF FOR A SHORT WHILE; BUT THE OUTCOME OF BIRTH REMAINS WITH THE PARENTS AND THE CHILD FOR LIFE.

WHO BENEFITS FROM ALTERNATIVES? No one wants to do something that does not benefit him or her in some way. So let's look at who could benefit from alternatives in childbirth. It could be everyone concerned. First, parents benefit. Parents must be considered first since the birth process affects them directly, first and foremost. No matter how we look at birth, the responsibility of birth remains with the parents all of their lives. The outcome of birth is only in the hands of the obstetrician and the hospital staff for a short while. But the outcome of birth remains with the parents and the child for life. Alternatives in childbirth force parents to make a positive choice. In so doing, they are obviously assuming some of the responsibility of their choice. Assuming responsibility in the choice in birth carries over into parenting. It follows, then, that when parents have assumed more responsibility for birth they will also be more responsible parents.

Second, doctors benefit. Doctors are very busy. Hard work. Difficult hours. A great amount of responsibility. These are all the reasons given for *less* personal care prenatally and during labor and birth. With more midwives and specially trained people to help with prenatal care and to attend normal birth in the *hospital, in child-bearing centers, and at home,* this would free the highly trained obstetricians to concentrate on the aspects of birth in which their training has also been concentrated. Furthermore, alternative birth choices place more responsibility on parents and less on doctors-- thus lessening the proneness to malpractice suits.

DOCTORS WOULD BENEFIT FROM ALTERNATIVES BECAUSE SUCH CHOICES PLACE MORE RESPONSIBILITY ON PARENTS AND LESS ON THEM, THUS LESSENING THE PRONENESS TO MALPRACTICE SUITS.

Third, midwives benefit. Alternatives would of necessity include more midwives than are now being used. They are uniquely trained to handle normal pregnancy, labor, and birth. They would work with laboring women in the normal births they enjoy and find exciting, freeing the obstetricians to deal with the complications and emergencies for which they have been trained.

It is my opinion that birth and birth procedures will never reflect what women want until women are in charge of birth.   It is strange to me that men have control of this uniquely womanly function. Women's sexuality is very much a part of pregnancy, childbirth, and lactation. Could women better understand men's sexual function than a man? I think not. Neither do I think that men understand women's sexual function better than women. No matter how sympathetic a man may be, he will never know the experience of childbirth.

Fourth, hospitals benefit. Sound homebirth programs and child-bearing centers would gradually move most births out of the hospitals, thus freeing much needed hospital beds for really sick patients who need the space. We have been told that obstetrics usually loses money for the hospital. If this is so, the hospital administration should be happy to let normal birth take place elsewhere.

Fifth, the public at large benefits. First, as costs go up, I think it is being shown that good homebirth programs and childbearing centers can provide better programs for less money. Everyone is concerned about the high cost of health care. I have noticed that many committees are being formed to explore the reasons for this and to come up with solutions. I think that birth alternatives should be explored regarding the cost aspect of health care.

Now I would like to philosophize a bit. I think that the improvement of birth, making it more family oriented and positive, will benefit society at large. I think that many of our problems of society today reflect the practice of separating families at birth. Marshall Klaus has done some remarkable studies showing the long reaching positive effects of early and close mother-infant contact, as opposed to the negative long-range effects of separation of mother and infant at birth. If this is true, is it any wonder that fathers who have had no contact with their baby for several days, except to view them through glass in the nursery, have trouble relating to their children at all?

I THINK THAT MANY OF OUR PROBLEMS OF SOCIETY TODAY REFLECT THE PRACTICE OF SEPARATING FAMILIES AT BIRTH.

Just look at the separatist point of view that Americans take. There are adult functions and there are children functions and never the twain shall meet. Of course, all functions cannot be family functions. There is a place for segregated activities. Today's conference is an example of a necessary and primarily adult function. But that doesn't mean our babies are not welcome. We have five children with us, but not all here in this room. How many parents, even though they feel it is the right thing to do, have the courage to bring a baby to an adult party or even to some restaurants, for that matter. How many big brothers want to include their little brothers and sisters in their play? We are always segregating people agewise. Perhaps a culmination of this separatist policy is the growing number of old folks homes, and even old folks cities.

Could the lack of imprinting and parent-child bonding at birth be reflected in the rising crime rate, in teenage rebellion? We don't know, but we should ask ourselves these questions. When you stop and think about it, it is not as farfetched as it may sound. We think that *Safe Alternatives in Childbirth* is a powerful idea that can positively affect our whole lives and the lives of our children which, in turn, would create a better world of living for all.

MATERNITY PRACTICES AROUND THE WORLD: HOW DO WE MEASURE UP?

Doris Haire, DMS*

Nowhere on earth is childbirth more distorted and warped than in the United States. In the effort to organize and streamline human parturition to the *convenience* of the American physician, the nurse midwife, the nursing staff, and the scientist so they only have to park once a day, we have allowed childbirth to be stripped of its magnificent power, its awesome beauty, its dignity, and its potential for growth for both the health professional and the parents.

Babies born in American hospitals are routinely subjected to an *environmental onslaught* before and after birth that would make the average Dutch obstetrician or health professional cringe in fright. Of all the countries I have visited, and I have visited 36 countries, to observe obstetric practices and visit maternity facilities, I am absolutely convinced that the United States has to be the most bizzarre country on earth in its management of obstetrics.

Because the majority of Dutch mothers still give birth at home or in a small maternity hospital attended by midwives, Dutch physicians, midwives, and nurses are exposed and imbued during their training with an appreciation of the important biological checks and balances organized by nature to assure the normal progress of labor and birth and to assure an optimal outcome for the baby. In general, the Dutch intervene in the birth process only when nature fails or falters.

In contrast, intervention in the normal progress of labor and birth in the United States is not only permitted, it is encouraged by our system of training. The typical American health professional completes his or her education and training without ever having witnessed a single truly normal labor and birth.

The thought of watching a woman in labor eating a light meal in the labor lounge or walking about the hospital grounds with her husband after she has checked into the hospital would cause most American health professionals to grow faint. I had one doctor who said that he "would really like to try out what normal childbirth could do for a mother." I said, "Okay. The first thing is you let her eat." And he went ashen. So that did that. We don't know the long term effects, or even the short term effects, of not permitting mothers to eat normally when in labor.

---

* *DORIS HAIRE is President of the American Foundation of Maternal and Child Health; Former President of the International Childbirth Education Association (ICEA), Current Member of the Board of ICEA and ICEA Representative to the U.S. Department of Health, Education and Welfare and the Federal Food and Drug Administration; Coauthor, with her husband, John, of the book, "Implementing Family Centered Maternity Care," and author of "The Cultural Warping of Childbirth," "Childbirth in the Netherlands: A Contrast in Care," and numerous other works.*

BABIES BORN IN AMERICAN HOSPITALS ARE ROUTINELY SUBJECTED TO AN ENVIRONMENTAL ONSLAUGHT BEFORE AND AFTER BIRTH THAT WOULD MAKE THE AVERAGE DUTCH HEALTH PROFESSIONAL CRINGE IN FRIGHT.

For the last ten years I have traveled about the United States lecturing to the hospital personnel on the importance of creating a home-like environment for the couple experiencing childbirth in the hospital. I have seen many improvements. Labor lounges are popping up everywhere. Mothers are being delivered in their labor beds and children are now allowed to visit their mothers in the hospital. But these practices are still exceptions, and the exceptions are rare. I, for one, will continue to work to improve hospital maternity, for there will still be mothers for years to come who will deliver in the hospital, especially those who are at risk.

But my ten years' experience has convinced me that American maternity care is frequently detrimental and often destructive. If we are to produce a normal generation of children with normal intelligence we must begin now to find safe alternatives in childbirth for low risk mothers and their babies in order that they will not become high risk as a result of their care in the hospital.

OF ALL THE 36 COUNTRIES I HAVE VISITED TO OBSERVE MATERNITY FACILITIES, I AM ABSOLUTELY CONVINCED THAT THE UNITED STATES HAS TO BE THE MOST BIZARRE ON EARTH IN ITS MANAGEMENT OF OBSTETRICS.

The impact of this conference, and I feel this very strongly, is likely to be felt around the world, if not today, then later, for the rest of the world follows us. No matter what we seem to do, the rest of the world tries to catch up whether it is good or bad. So I feel that this meeting today will have a tremendous impact on maternity care around the world.

As I look upon this audience today, I am filled with a sense of pride. I am proud of you who dare to challenge this unscientific tradition of "American obstetric care." I am proud of you who dare to pioneer in order to find safe alternatives in childbirth despite the pressure from established institutions. And I would like to say a special word for Ruth Lubic, Director of the Maternity Center Association in New York City, a newly reorganized childbearing center which has been the target of vigorous opposition from the NY District of the American College of Obstetricians & Gynecologists, because no one in this world has been more harassed as far as I am concerned and I think that she is a very noble person among Americans.

IT IS A COMMENT ON OUR TIMES THAT WE, WHO MERELY WANT TO INCLUDE THE LOVE AND TENDERNESS OF ONE'S FAMILY IN CHILDBIRTH, ARE CONSIDERED RADICALS.

It is a comment on our times that we, who want childbirth to again become an intimate family affair, filled with the security of one's home and the love and tenderness of one's family, are considered radicals. Some of you may be here today because you are curious, but most of you are here because you are concerned with the aggressive, pathological management of hospital based obstetric care in the U.S. and are seeking safe alternatives.

The late Rachael Carson, who was also concerned with the adverse effects of technology, wrote these words many years ago and I quote: "The 'control of nature' is a phrase conceived in arrogance, born of a Neanderthal age of biology and philosophy when it was supposed that nature exists for the convenience of man." Surely our present form of obstetric care in the U.S. is conceived in arrogance and born of a Neanderthal age of biology and philosophy.

AMERICAN MATERNITY CARE IS FREQUENTLY DETRIMENTAL AND OFTEN DESTRUCTIVE. IF WE ARE TO PRODUCE A NORMAL GENERATION OF CHILDREN WITH NORMAL INTELLIGENCE WE MUST BEGIN NOW TO FIND SAFE ALTERNATIVES IN CHILDBIRTH FOR LOW RISK MOTHERS IN ORDER THAT THEY WILL NOT BECOME HIGH RISK AS A RESULT OF THE HOSPITAL.

Most of the world's women give birth at home or in a small maternity home attended by a midwife; yet there is a drive in the U.S. to eliminate small obstetric units and consolidate American obstetric services in order to justify the high cost of expensively equipped and staffed intensive care units. The forcing of all women into large impersonal obstetric units is just one more example of the American penchant for adapting the entire system to meet the needs of the exceptions rather than the needs of the majority.

While we are told of the value of eliminating small and medium sized obstetric services, we find that a national survey of the U.S. carried out by the American College of Obstetricians and Gynecologists reveals that, in general, the larger the obstetric service the greater the rate of maternal and infant death. The survey also showed that the closer the affiliation between the obstetric service and a medical school, the greater the number of maternal and infant deaths. Undoubtedly, some of these deaths result from the fact that there was a greater incidence of high risk mothers in the larger teaching hospitals. But it is also possible that the greater tendency to intervene in the normal progress of labor and birth in these institutions to provide research and teaching opportunities for students, interns, and residents may contribute to these statistics and may also result in a disproportionately high incidence of our neurologically impaired children among full term, low risk mothers.

MOST DOCTORS WILL ADMIT THAT "IATROGENIA", WHICH IS "PHYSICIAN-CAUSED DISEASE OR DAMAGE", UNDOUBTEDLY CONTRIBUTES TO A LARGE PROPORTION OF OBSTETRIC COMPLICATIONS AND EMERGENCY SITUATIONS.

Now we must defend our country in one way--in that the U.S. is not alone in its pathological approach to obstetrics. I have been simply horrified by what I have seen abroad recently, in particular, the changes I have seen come about in England and Sweden. I saw babies so blue in Sweden last summer that I was frightened by the color and midwives in Sweden are now pushing epidurals because it is easier for the midwife. So there is no magic key and there is no time that we can ever relax and let the system roll on.

There are many obstetricians of renown who share our concern with the world trend toward pathologically oriented obstetrics. At a recent conference in New York sponsored by the American Foundation of Maternal and Child Health, Dr. Roberto Caldero-Barcia made the following statement, and I quote: "In the last forty years, many artificial practices have been introduced which have changed labor and birth from a physiological event to a very complicated, medical procedure in which all kinds of drugs and maneuvers are done, sometimes unnecessarily, and many of them potentially damaging to the baby and even for the mother." These are not the overly cautious words of an unsophisticated physician. In October of this year, Dr. Roberto Caldeyro-Barcia who is a world renowned scientist, will become the President of the International Federation of Gynecologists and Obstetricians. Unfortunately, the pathological approach to obstetrics, perfected in the U.S., is taking hold in other developed countries. I particularly saw this in Sweden and England.

THE VAST MAJORITY OF WOMEN ARE CAPABLE OF COMPLETELY NORMAL CHILDBIRTH AND CAN SAFELY GIVE BIRTH AT HOME.

It is interesting to note that in Great Britain, in their perinatal statistics, the lowest incidence of infant deaths was among babies delivered at home by professional midwives. Not *nurse midwives*, but *professional midwives*. I would like to see us develop a program in this country for professional midwives. In many countries they feel that this is a very important way to go. Dr. Kloosterman of the Netherlands feels strongly about this. He is a highly respected obstetrician from the University of Amsterdam.

IN GREAT BRITAIN THE LOWEST INCIDENCE OF INFANT DEATH HAS BEEN FOUND TO BE AMONG BABIES DELIVERED AT HOME BY PROFESSIONAL MIDWIVES. NOT NURSE MIDWIVES, BUT PROFESSIONAL MIDWIVES.

Among the many obstetric practices Dr. Caldeyro-Barcia cited as potentially dangerous to both mother and baby were:
* Routine artificial rupture of embryonic membranes
* Use of uterine stimulants to start and accelerate labor without medical indication
* Prohibiting the mother from walking during labor
* Routine use of drugs rather than providing strong emotional support to relieve the mother's distress
* And placing the mother on her back during labor and birth.

Despite these strong statements by one of the world's most respected obstetricians, the interesting thing is that I have been in several university centers lately and every single mother I have seen in the last six months has been flat on her back. What are the students and faculty reading at these universities? I mean, who is reading *this* material? Sometimes I think we are the only ones who are bothering to read it.

I might say, here, that it is terribly important that you read the scientific literature. For us to have feelings is nothing. What we have to have is references. So don't underestimate the power of scientific discussion. If you are going to play with the big fellows, you have got to play by their rules.

In Dr. Caldeyro-Barcia's institution at Montevideo, and the Montevidean population is primarily European in background, not South American Indian, they have reduced the incidence of *medication* from 100% to only 10% and this is in an institution where 60% of the mothers are high risk. Despite the warnings of Caldeyro-Barcia and others, few hospital based obstetricians have changed their traditional role or traditional mode of obstetrics. As a result, American parents have become increasingly distrustful of hospital based obstetric care and are beginning to opt for childbirth at home surrounded by friends, family, and familiar surroundings.

PARENTS MUST BEGIN TO DEMAND FROM OBSTETRICIANS TO PROVE THAT WHAT THEY ARE DOING IS SAFE. IF THEY CHALLENGE YOU ABOUT BIRTHS AT HOME OR OTHER ALTERNATIVES, YOU MUST DEMAND THAT THEY PROVE TO YOU THAT THEIR METHOD IS BETTER.

At home light tasks help to keep the couple occupied during the long hours of labor. I can't help but think how funny it is that we have had to devise an abnormal type of breathing to distract the mother when doing the dishes or dusting would probably be far better.

The vast majority of women are capable of completely normal childbirth and can safely give birth at home. However, the present trend towards homebirth should not cloud the fact that the hospital is clearly the safest place for childbirth for those childbearing women who are at risk, women with identified diseases such as heart disease, diabetes, toxemia, and other adverse conditions such as maternal-fetal blood incompatibility, premature labor or prolonged gestation. In these instances of high risk, survival of a vulnerable mother and baby is far more likely to be in a hospital equipped with an intensive care unit for both.

But is the hospital the safest place for a healthy childbearing woman who has been found to have no adverse conditions during her prenatal visits? In theory, the hospital should be the safest environment for birth for all women. But is it?

Physicians frequently consider parents who opt for a homebirth to be reckless and irresponsible because, they say, 50-60% of all complications which occur during labor and birth and the immediate postpartum period occur among obstetric patients who give no indications of being at risk during pregnancy. This seems to be a *damning defense* of the present system of obstetric care. It compels one to ask what proportion of these complications, which had their onset *during* labor and birth, are the direct result of aggressive obstetric procedures carried out in the hospital for a variety of non-medical reasons. Among these reasons would be: (1) To start or speed up the mother's labor for either the convenience of the doctor or the mother or both; (2) To keep the mother comfortable even at the expense of jeopardizing the integrity of the fetal brain; or (3) To provide a learning experience for medical students, interns, and residents.

Professor G.J. Kloosterman, Chairman of the Department of Obstetrics at the University of Amsterdam, has stated repeatedly that the spontaneous labor in a healthy woman is an event marked by a number of processes which are so complex and so perfectly attuned to each other that any interference will *only* distract from their optimal character. The doctor, always on the lookout for pathology and eager to interfere, will much too often change true physiologic aspects of human reproduction into pathology. Now, this is a doctor speaking who may well be the next President of the International Federation of Gynecologists and Obstetricians. He has already been nominated once. So these are learned men who feel that labor is best left to nature unless nature falters.

There is no question that American expertise has saved tens of thousands of lives over the years. However, most doctors will admit that "iatrogenia," which is "physician-caused disease or damage," undoubtedly contributes to a large proportion of obstetric complications and emergency situations. By the way, there is an excellent paper on that that just came out in Lancet. I think it is April 10th, Lancet, called "Obstetric Care Today--For Better or For Worse?" It's a very humorous and very frightening paper at the same time.

The administration of drugs to relieve the mother's apprehension and discomfort during pregnancy, labor, and birth, and the use of Pitocin and other oxytocic drugs to induce or stimulate the uterus in order to speed up labor are just two examples of obstetric intervention which upset the normal, bio-physiological checks and balances nature has organized to regulate normal birth. Such interference is now routine in many obstetric hospital units in the U.S. and such intervention would be frowned upon in the Netherlands. Now, I say the Netherlands because there are still hospitals in Sweden and in Europe where normal childbirth occurs, but tragically the number is being reduced every day. Only in the Netherlands can you still find babies that are reasonably "untouched by human hands," so to speak.

There is no question that the welfare of their patients has always been the deep concern of American physicians, nurse midwives, and nurses. The unphysiologic practices which have become so much a part of American obstetric care to the point that such practices have become accepted as the norm appear to have gradually been built up as a result of social customs and cultural patterning. But cultural patterning can be changed and *must* be changed.

Dr. Jerold Lucey, who was then Chairman of the Committee on the Fetus and the Newborn of the American Academy of Pediatrics, changed my whole direction a few years ago when he said to me, "Doris, you're wasting your time trying to convince obstetricians that what you want is right. You parents must begin to demand from obstetricians to prove to you that what they are doing is safe." That is what you should all be doing in my opinion. If they challenge you about your births at home or in other alternative programs, you must demand that they prove to you that their method is better.

This was the turning point in my life. It was the end of my frustration because I found that there was virtually no scientific support for almost any obstetric procedure carried out for a healthy parturient.
    * There is no scientific support for separating the mother from her family during labor and birth.
    * There is no scientific support for routine medication and it's important that you realize that the American Academy of Pediatrics Committee on Drugs has stated that "there is no drug that has been proven safe for the unborn child." I think that was one of the most noble statements that ever came out of the Academy of Pediatrics. I'm sure there was tremendous pressure on the academy once it was said. It has been of tremendous value to parents and I am proud of them.
    * There is no scientific support for shaving the perineum. You probably all know that Burchell, Ob & Gyn, 24:272-273, 1964, and Kantor, Ob & Gyn, 25:509-512, 1965, have both found that it actually increases the incidence of infection.
    * There is no scientific support for the routine electronic monitoring of the fetus. It has not been shown to reduce neurologic impairment in children.
    * Ultrasound. I talked to Dr. Yen, who is the Head of the Bureau of Medical Devices, and she told me that her Bureau is extremely concerned about the long term delayed effects of ultrasound. No one has done a scientifically controlled study. There are two studies going on now, one in England and one in Canada, but they are only four years old.
    * X-rays. I am old enough (50 in case you want to know) that I have friends now who have cancer as a result of X-ray therapy for acne, thyroid, and tonsils. Cancer is coming up among young dentists who were practicing on each other in dental school for dental X-rays. At the time this was considered a perfectly safe therapy. So what are we doing exposing millions of American children, unborn children, to procedures for which no one knows the long term effects?
    * There is no scientific support for rupturing the amniotic membranes and Caldeyro-Barcia has shown this very clearly through x-ray photography and other ways, that this creates stress for the fetal head.
    * There is no scientific justification for routine episiotomy. I cannot stress enough that *there is no scientific support* in any country of the world or from any health agency in the world that shows any health advantage to routine episiotomy and I get darn tired of seeing it in all the obstetric textbooks as if it were God's word.
    * Stirrups. I dream of the day when putting a woman's legs in stirrups when there is no medical indication will be considered malpractice.

    * Pregnant women in the United States are seldom advised that
many of the obstetric related drugs such as uterine stimulants, spi-
nals, paracervical blocks, and epidurals can interfere with the transfer of oxygen from the mother's bloodstream to her unborn baby and
his brain. It is important that you realize that no one knows the
degree of oxygen deprivation an unborn or newborn infant can tolerate
before he or she sustains permanent brain damage.

    It is likely that most American women would not be so quick to
demand pharmocalogic relief from their discomfort if they were advised of the potential dangers of the drugs to the integrity of their
baby's brain and its future intellectual functioning. There is no
doubt in my mind that obstetric drugs contribute to the skyrocketing
incidence of learning disabilities in the United States and that
alternatives to our present system would reduce this incidence.

THE AMERICAN ACADEMY OF PEDIATRICS HAS STATED THAT
"THERE IS NO DRUG THAT HAS BEEN PROVEN SAFE FOR
THE UNBORN CHILD."

    I met all day yesterday at the Food and Drug Administration
with heads of pharmaceutical industries and the industry representatives and the heads of pharmacists' organizations of this country. It
was interesting. The pharmacists were very much for telling the patients that the long term effects of the drugs were not known, but
the one thing the pharmaceutical industry resisted was a statement
that I would like to have put in the patient label or package insert
that says, "It is important that you understand that the long term
effects or delayed effects of this drug are unknown." On that one
thing they balked--absolutely terrified with the idea.

    Despite the potential danger maternal hypotension poses to
the fetal brain, a drop in maternal blood pressure resulting from
obstetric drugs has become so common among American obstetric patients
that in many instances it is not even noted on the mother's labor
and delivery chart--unless it is a significant drop. But we must ask:
"What is a *significant* drop in maternal blood pressure?" Unfortunately,
no one knows. Scientists have had a fairly good idea of how the
mother would be affected by the various degrees of hypotension but no
one knows how much a drop in maternal blood pressure can occur before
the transfer of oxygen from the mother to the fetus is so reduced that
the fetal brain is permanently damaged. A vasopressin drug can be
administered to the mother to increase her blood pressure, but there
is absolutely no assurance that the blood flow to the uterus will
return to normal quickly enough to avoid damage to the fetal brain.

    I think it is important, again, that you know that the research
coming out indicates that the electronic fetal monitor cannot tell the
onset of effects to the fetal brain because the fetal brain is affected
at least 15 minutes *before* it shows up on the fetal heartrate monitor.
They are doing electroencephalograms (EEGs) on babies to show this.
Again, they have to rupture the membranes to do it, but if they're
going to rupture them, they may as well find something important.

MOTHER'S ARMS ARE, BY FAR, THE SAFEST BABY WARMER THAT HAS EVER BEEN INVENTED.

Dutch infants born in the hospital spend most of the first hours of life cuddled warmly in their alert mother's arms and, I might say, the mother's arms are, by far, the safest baby warmer that has ever been invented. I heard a lecture by a fellow who is head of a company who tests electronic hospital material and I was simply appalled by the things that can go wrong with an electronic hospital baby warmer. So don't let the baby out of your sight if it is in one of those baby warmers. One of the things they mentioned was that when they raise the baby up to measure it, it burns the baby's feet. The thermistor can also become detached. Now, these are all human errors and human errors are forgivable. But, then on the other hand, if the mother is alert and in reasonably good condition, why not put the baby in the mother's arms?

Blue hands and feet are seen so frequently among American hospital born infants after the first *hour* of life that parents are now being told that such a condition is normal. In commenting on the frequency of this condition among American newborn infants, Dr. Albert Huch, obstetrician-physiologist for the University of Marburg, Germany, recently said at Dartmouth College, "You Americans consider blue hands and feet after the first minutes of life to be normal. But we do not consider a baby in that condition to be in optimal condition." Therein lies the difference.

American physicians and many parents have, in general, begun to accept the *average* baby's condition as *normal*, the best we can do. In the Netherlands, where more than half the babies are still delivered by a midwife in the mother's home or in a maternity home, the most striking difference can be seen in the robust color of the newborn infant. Fingers and toes of the Dutch newborn infant turn pink within seconds. Also, meconium staining is the result of a condition indicating fetal stress and is a common happening in American hospitals while it is considered a sign of danger in other countries. We here today want our babies to be born in *optimal* condition, not merely average.

THE FDA DOES NOT REQUIRE A PHYSICIAN TO REPORT AN ADVERSE DRUG REACTION. NEITHER DOES THE FDA GUARANTEE THE SAFETY OF ANY DRUG, NOT EVEN THOSE THE AGENCY RELEASES AND APPROVES AS "SAFE AND EFFECTIVE."

Another thing that is important for you to realize is that the U.S. Food and Drug Administration does not require all manufacturers of obstetric related drugs to carry out scientifically controlled long term follow-ups on children exposed to the various drugs in utero to determine if there are any delayed, adverse effects on later neurologic development. I think that is a particularly interesting fact because one of the representatives of a major drug manufacturing company said yesterday that this *was* required. So if he doesn't know this, we are really in trouble.

The FDA does not require a physician to report an adverse drug reaction to the FDA. I also have a letter from Richard Crowd who is Director of the FDA Bureau of Drugs stating: "The FDA does not guarantee the safety of any drug, not even those the agency releases or approves as safe and effective."

One in every 35 children born in the United States today will eventually be diagnosed as retarded according to the National Association of Retarded Children. In 75% of these cases, there is no genetic or familial predisposing factor. At least one out of 17 children, and in some very upper-class areas it is as high as one in 4 or 5, born in the United States has been found to have some form of learning disability or dysfunction. I called the Superintendent of Schools at Grosse Point, Michigan, which is where Henry Ford and all the lovely people live, and one out of every 10 children in Grosse Point is in a special class. Now, they don't call them "learning disabled." They just put them in reading therapy or something special like that. In Scarsdale, New York, one out of 4 or 5 children are in such classes. In Phoenix, Arizona, in the best neighborhoods, it is also one out of 4 or 5. What are we doing with our hospital maternity care? It is obvious that we have to find safer alternatives. The product we are producing with our present form of obstetric care is not good enough.

I, for one, will continue to work for well organized, professionally attended homebirth services such as that found in the Netherlands for I am convinced that domiciliary obstetric service for low risk mothers and babies will free hospitals to give really excellent indepth care to high risk mothers. Such a homebirth service will return childbirth to the realm of a normal physiologic experience, will prevent meddlesome obstetrics, and will provide educational experiences for future nurses and physicians which will prepare them to understand the intricate checks and balances comprising normal parturition. The Dutch have taught us that a well organized domiciliary obstetric service has been shown to be safe and is clearly within our reach. I call upon the medical establishment and the government to show some imagination and to spend less money on bureaucratic empires and more money on funding *Safe Alternatives in Childbirth*.

EDITORS' NOTE: Scientific documentation for many of the statements made here by Dr. Haire is contained in her publication,"The Cultural Warping of Childbirth," which cites more than 100 papers from medical journals. It is available for $1.60 from the ICEA Supplies Center, P.O. Box 70258, Seattle, Washington 98107. Documentation of many of Dr. Haire's statements is also contained in the article by Frederic M. Ettner, MD, found later in this book in the Chapter entitled: Study of Obstetrics: 1975, pp. 37-66.

CHILDBEARING & MATERNITY CENTERS - ALTERNATIVES TO HOMEBIRTH & HOSPITAL

Betty Hosford, RN, CNM, & Ruth Watson Lubic, RN, CNM

Maternity Center Association's Childbearing Center in New York was born as a result of the Childbirth Revolution, first noticed by us in 1970, and was organized for the express purpose of offering a safe alternative to those parents who, for a variety of reasons, opt out of the system and choose homebirth--do-it-yourself maternity care.

The Childbearing Center is a demonstration project - designed to test a possible solution to the problem evidenced by disenchantment of a growing number of parents with traditional obstetrical care. It is committed to several large objectives.

1. To offer true alternatives in care- The "Half-Way House" set up to embrace as many features of homebirth as possible with carefully built-in safety features - and to simulate hospital in regard to emergency equipment - to greatest possible degree. For example, we have an ambulance service which can effect transfer to our back-up hospital in eleven minutes. We have oxygen, intravenous capability, blood volume expanders, emergency drugs and infant resuscitation equipment.

2. To offer care which is planned with and for parents according to individual needs and wishes -- the Center is designed for parents who wish to take a more responsible role in health care -- there are no "routines." A discussion of labor plans is conducted with each family. Families are very much a part of the decision making team providing care. For example, desires regarding position at delivery -- where to spend labor -- necessity for episiotomy, etc. -- are all considered individually. Many of our parents are "with" Leboyer.

3. To provide a strong educational component - this objective is a most important one for many reasons:
   * It provides an orientation toward health education in general, preparation for parenthood is stressed, based on belief that the maternity cycle offers a most unique and significant opportunity to influence health and promote preventive medicine in the future.
   * Nutrition, health, hygiene, as well as all physical and psychological aspects of childbearing are stressed -- one major goal being to help parents become more proficient in physical assessment of family members and in assumption of a more active role in their own health care.
   * The educational component also provides parents an opportunity to make *informed* choices - whether about infant feeding, circumcision, or how to select a pediatrician.

---

* BETTY HOSFORD is Coordinator, Maternity Center Association, New York City; and Educational Director for Nurse Midwifery Internship, Downstate Medical Center, Brooklyn, New York.

* RUTH WATSON LUBIC is General Director and Assistant Secretary, Maternity Center Association, New York City; A former Officer in the American College of Nurse Midwives; Member of Board of Consultants, International Childbirth Education Association; and Charter Member of the Institute of Medicine, National Academy of Science..

* Education helps the "low risk" families eligible for care at the Center become even *more low risk* by affording them the opportunity to come to labor and birth in excellent physical condition and nutrition.
* The educational component also is designed to prepare families for early discharge by helping them to understand in depth the physical and psychological changes of the post-partum and early parenting period and their significance.

In the words of one parent - "The greatest thing about the experience was that we came home with a growing feeling of confidence."

4. A fourth objective of the Childbearing Center is to provide low cost quality maternity care. The CbC's "Package" is about 1/3 to 1/4 that of private hospital rates in New York. For example, in one tertiary hospital in New York, with the labor, delivery and three day post-partum fee at $1,300, obstetrical fee for delivery only at $700, and each pre- and post-natal visit at $30, the entire cost can easily amount to $2,300 plus.

5. Very important to the Center Staff also is the provision of personalized, meticulously implemented antepartum care. We aim for 38-40% hematocrit, for example, to insure optimum physical health and positive emotional outlook of mothers.

What are the advantages of birth in the Maternity Center as identified by parents to date?
"More personalized care"
"The closest thing to home away from home"
"Having baby with you every minute"
"So peaceful and relaxed"
These are but a few of the positive responses we have received.

BIRTH IN THE CENTER IS TRULY A CELEBRATION FOR THE STAFF IN SEEING BIRTH IN THE PERSPECTIVE OF A JOYOUS SIGNIFICANT FAMILY EXPERIENCE WITH ROUTINES AND PROCEDURES BECOMING SECONDARY FOR WHAT, TO THE FAMILY, IS THE "EXPERIENCE OF A LIFETIME." AND, ALL WITHIN THE FRAMEWORK OF A PRIORITY FOR SAFETY TOO.

Some of the *subtle* but *definite* built-in safety features include:

1. The emphasis on nutrition and health which brings mother and baby to labor and delivery in best possible condition to weather all stresses.
2. Caloric and fluid intake during labor to protect mother, and especially baby, from hazards of acidosis or near acidosis, for which we are ever alert.
3. Walking and sitting during labor and an upright delivery position to provide baby an opportunity for 100% oxygenation.
4. The homelike surroundings with support which provide the *least* stressful atmosphere and promote greatest ease of labor. To date no analgesics have been needed for labor - with the exception of only one mother to whom Demerol was given for lack of progress, to rest her rather than relieve stress.

> WE AIM FOR "APGAR TWELVE" BABIES. OUR TWO EXTRA
> UNOFFICIAL POINTS COME FROM (1) PINK TO THE TOENAILS
> AT MOMENT OF BIRTH AND (2) ONE EXTRA POINT IF THE BABY CRIES
> BEFORE BEING COMPLETELY BORN.

5. The mother in control provides another safety feature: We aim for "Apgar Twelve" babies -- and encourage mother to do much deep breathing around time of birth so she can literally flood her circulation with oxygen and make it available to baby. Our two extra unofficial points come from (a) pink to toenails at moment of birth and (b) one extra point to the baby if he cries before he's all born.

6. A sixth **safety** feature is early breastfeeding and/or bonding. Babies feed frequently from birth on. Most of them apparently have not read the book and, instead of getting drowsy after an hour, tend to nip and nap for 2-3 or more. One of the most recent babies nursed and drowsed off and on for 5 hours. Needless to say, his milk supply was in the very next day! The atmosphere is set, too, for helping mother and father to fall in love with the baby. Results of this early contact are evident in our babies *weight gain* who average 1/2 pound *over* birth weight at 6-7 days. One cherub distinguished herself by being 9 ounces over in 5 days!

7. Visiting nurse follow-up is a vital safety aspect of the program. They report responsible, outstanding relationships between parents and babies. We observed one father and his 5 1/2 week old "talking" to one another at the time of mother's post-partum check-up.

Only time will tell what all this means.

> THERE HAS NEVER BEEN FOUND BY US, OR PRESENTED TO US,
> ANY EVIDENCE THAT DEMONSTRATES OUR CENTER'S PLACEMENT
> OUT-OF-HOSPITAL WILL, IN AND OF ITSELF, CAUSE IT TO BE UNSAFE.

We have learned by experience of two important areas for concentration:

1. Parents fear "risk out." The subject of alternative plans in the event the family becomes ineligible for the Center before birth must be carefully interpreted and followed up.

2. Carefully planned pediatric and obstetrical follow-up care is another must which cannot be overemphasized.

What kind of effect has the program had on the professionals who function in it? Birth at the Center is truly a celebration. For the staff there is great joy in seeing birth in the perspective of a wonderfully joyous, significant family experience with routines and procedures becoming secondary for what, to the family, is the "experience of a lifetime." All within the framework of a priority for safety, of course.

Having shared with you some perceptions from the point of view of families and clinicians, we would like now to explore with you some of the areas on which we are most often questioned by curious visitors. Frequently asked is, "Why not home delivery?" MCA considered a return to home delivery and rejected the idea for two reasons:

1. In our experience the systematized home delivery service is not inexpensive. During the course of our development of the Childbearing Center, Dr. Louis Hellman in conversation suggested that we consider the possibility of a return to home delivery. I raised the question of the cost of providing such a service, particularly when the size of the professional staff necessary to adequately cover the needs of such a service is considered. He recalled that at the time Johns-Hopkins closed its delivery service in the mid 50's, the cost was considered to be about $800 per patient. Although at Maternity Center we charged $10 to families enrolling in our home delivery service, the cost, of course, was much higher.

2. There was a second factor in our thinking. Even prior to the time we closed our homebirth service in 1958 it had begun to be unsafe for our staff to be on the streets of New York at all hours. We had instituted a plan in which a family member met the nurse-midwife and escorted her to the home of the parturient. At that time we were trying to meet the needs of families of small means native both outside and inside the U.S. who were either unused to utilizing the hospital or afraid of it.

The Maternity Center Association Childbearing Center opened in September, 1975, after 2.5 years of development and the securing from New York State of *all* legal and regulatory permissions, which was no easy job. Included were review by 3 advisory agencies peopled by providers and consumers. We are Blue Cross approved and Medicaid eligible; the City of New York, however, has refused to issue the Center a Medicaid vendor number thus delaying reimbursement and, effectively, denying our personalized, family centered care to low income families. We operate under New York State law as a Diagnostic and Treatment Center, not as an adaptation of a hospital. The Center has the strong support of prestigious physicians such as Philip R. Lee, MD, Assistant Secretary for Health in the L.B. Johnson administration. Nevertheless it is opposed by some individual physicians and by the local district of the ACOG which, in a recent position paper, *overtly* objects to all out-of-hospital placement on the ground of safety. The Commissioner of Health of the City of New York, on the advice of his obstetrical advisory committee, also disapproves. Perhaps, therefore, it is pertinent to share with you the reasons why we place it in our town house on East 92nd Street.

1. We are trying to bring back into "the system" those families "opting out" for do-it-yourself home delivery. They are deeply alienated from hospitals.
2. We want to "cost" the project carefully. It is virtually impossible to do this in an acute care hospital setting.
3. We are trying to develop a model which will have utility in under-served areas--both urban and rural.

4. The biases of hospital personnel and staff often make it difficult to develop such innovations within a hospital setting.

5. In teaching centers, the demand for student physician educational experience can take priority over fulfilling promises made to childbearing families.

6. The State of New York's Public Health Council gave its permission to implement the project in the time, at the place, and in the manner described and no other.

Finally, there has never been found by us, or presented to us, any evidence that demonstrates our Center's placement out-of-hospital will in and of itself cause it to be unsafe. As a matter of fact, our own 28 year experience with home delivery (1931-1959) and that of the Frontier Nursing Service, Chicago Maternity Center, and even the recent review of over 1,000 home deliveries in California by Lewis E. Mehl, MD, (see Mehl's article pp. 73-100 in this book) all suggest that a unit such as the Childbearing Center *will* provide safe care.

In any event, through the medium of a 4 page general consent and personal interview, families select us with *full* knowledge of the risks of childbearing in general and our means of handling problems should they arise. And, as you may well know, hospitals can introduce other risks such as those of potential infection and intervention.

Our unit is designed for healthy families expecting a normal birth and so couples seeking our care are screened very carefully. Care is provided by a team consisting of obstetricians, nurse-midwives, public health nurses, a pediatrician, and midwife assistants. Families receive all ante- and intrapartum care in the Center. They return home in up to 12 hours after delivery and are seen in their homes on the 1st and 3rd-5th day by Public Health Nurses. They return to us on the 6th or 7th day and again at the 5th to 6th week for the usual postpartum check. A pediatric exam is given the infant before discharge from the Center.

WITH THE ENCOURAGEMENT TO EARLY BREASTFEEDING AND CLOSE FAMILY CONTACT, THE ATMOSPHERE IS SET FOR HELPING MOTHER AND FATHER TO FALL IN LOVE WITH THEIR BABY. RESULTS OF THIS EARLY CONTACT ARE EVIDENT, EVEN ON MEDICAL-PHYSICAL GROUNDS, BY THE FACT THAT OUR BABIES AVERAGE HALF A POUND OVER BIRTH WEIGHT AT 6-7 DAYS.

The Childbearing Center is, as I have said, in a townhouse on East 92nd Street in New York and we invite you to come to see us. We run orientations three times a week: Wednesday mornings, Wednesday evenings, and Saturday afternoons. These orientations begin in what we call our "multipurpose" room which is also used for childcare and our parents classes. It was once the dining room of John Sloan and his wife.

The orientation is designed for parents. When a family calls us and says "We are interested in coming into your unit and becoming part of your unit" we *require* them to go through an orientation *before* they make up their minds about whether, in fact, they would like to give birth in our Center. At that orientation there is a tour given of the facilities. We explain all about us, what we have, what we do not have, what we feel the risks are, and we invite them to ask all kinds of questions. We get asked some pretty hard questions, too. But we feel that the establishment of trust is extremely important, particularly with families alienated from the system in general.

Following the orientation, even if families feel that at the moment they want to come with us, we ask them to go home and talk it over--with their family, with their gynecologist, with their physician, with their mother-in-law, their cousins, uncles, anybody. We want them to feel perfectly comfortable about coming to us. And if they do, after that time, decide they want to come in, then call for an appointment.

When they call, we then send them a packet of materials which includes the general consent that I mentioned, as well as their own history sheets which they fill out themselves. We feel that it is important for families to be involved in their own care. We try to make them feel that it is *their* history we are asking about and not our version as we would record it on paper. We also send them information about payment plans. They also receive a questionnaire so that we can know where they are in terms of knowledge and information about pregnancy and childbearing. A "Family Handbook" is included which reiterates information about the Center so that we are perfectly sure that families have, on a repeated basis, adequate information about us.

Regarding the nature of our actual facilities, we have discovered that it is very difficult to make an examining room "home-like." We have an examining room which we use for labor admission, but we also have what we call the "family room" designed for family to be together in early labor. We also encourage families to go out and visit the museum if they come in early labor.

If families want children to participate in the labor-delivery experience, we ask them to bring someone in who can sit the child. We do permit children to be in the labor-delivery area. We have had as many as two children present at the birth of a sibling. The children's reaction is that "it's just no sweat at all."

We have two labor-delivery rooms. One is done in blues and greens and the other is done in orange and yellow. The bed is a reconstructed hospital bed. We have drilled the frame so that we can put on a very simple sling stirrups if we need to for the repair of a laceration or the suturing of an episiotomy.

We have had about 20 births, to date. We have done some episiotomies, but always after discussing this with the family. Our primigravida rate is about 30% and so it makes 70% of our mothers multigravida.

The family stays together for the whole time it is in the unit. The baby never leaves the family. We find that the basinet is the least used piece of equipment in the room. A recliner is provided for the father.

The beds are high-low beds, but manually operated high-low beds. We have gotten special mattresses made for them. They are a firm foam mattress and are wider than the usual hospital mattress--approximately 3 inches wider, because we wanted mothers to feel comfortable with the baby on the bed with them, not like they were going to be falling off any minute. There are no side rails. Fathers are also permitted in the labor bed.

We are required to have sterilizing equipment by the State. We are also required to put in a heating, ventilating air conditioning unit which changes the air in the labor delivery room six times an hour. We culture constantly. We are very concerned about the possibility of infection because, unlike the home, we do have a variety of families using the unit. So we feel we need to be very careful.

We keep a clean utility room. In the "family room" families may stay there in their street clothes. But the labor-delivery room, the utility room, the kitchen, and the team station are considered to be "clean" and visitors must gown and change shoes to go these places.

We do encourage families to bring in their own food and if they have special teas they would like to drink, they are encouraged to bring them along. A refrigerator, stove, and sink are provided. We expect fathers to get up and fix for mothers if they are not too busy with support. There is some discussion about the beneficial distraction element of women washing dishes, etc., during labor. We don't discriminate against fathers washing dishes.

We ask families to bring in their own clean clothing to wear in labor and delivery. Even if a child is going to be present at labor-delivery we would expect families to bring a clean change of clothing for the child. In one instance we took in a rubber covered mat, like you would use for exercise practice with the preparation classes, and wiped it off carefully with antibacterial agents. The child was in there on that mat in the corner playing with toys which he had gotten used to from coming to classes there with his parents.

The pediatric exam is delayed as late as possible, until just before the family goes home. This gives the parents time to think of questions about the infant to pose to the pediatrician.

In conclusion, let me review how our families prepare and are prepared for parenting. We have not discussed the role that family life experiences play in determining any individual's commitment to and expectations regarding the parenting process. However, in the Childbearing Center we try to assist expectant parents to build on those experiences in order to develop self-confidence in their ability to bring forth and rear a child. We do this through a number of means:

1. Including parents as team members in decision making concerning their own care and that of the expected child.

2. Providing classes on all aspects of pregnancy, labor, delivery, and the newborn and its care.

3. Assisting families in selection of follow-up care to be initiated at appropriate times.

4. Providing a homelike emotionally supportive setting for the labor and delivery experience.

5. Welcoming support persons and/or family members to participate with the mother in the experience.

6. Providing the means for the family unit to remain together during the first hours of the infant's life.

7. During this period reinforcing the classroom teaching and encouraging families to demonstrate their knowledge of the infant's needs and the satisfaction of those needs.

8. Providing an evaluation of the infant by a teaching pediatrician.

9. Providing follow-up in the home by Public Health Nurses who have had an in-service program on the Center.

10. Making ourselves available to families at all times by telephone.

11. And offering opportunity for follow-up group sessions.

To·date, the experiences of families delivered in the Center have been gratifying. Visiting nurses are very impressed with the involvement and interaction of fathers as well as mothers with the infant. We are eager to institute an evaluation of the effects of our program on parenting. Perhaps the best test of all will be the future parenting behavior of the Childbearing Center babies themselves!

For More Information
On This Childbearing Center
Write:

MATERNITY CENTER ASSOCIATION
48 East 92nd Street
New York, NY 10028

Childbirth Alternatives and Infant Outcome: A Pediatric View

Robert S. Mendelsohn, MD, ACHO*

First, let us review the *conventional* attitudes on infant out-come in American Medicine. Second, questions will be raised regarding the *truth* of these conventional attitudes. And Third, *predictions* will be offered for the future.

CONVENTIONAL ATTITUDES

There is no better place for an infant to be born than in a modern hospital in the United States, staffed by board-certified obstetricians and pediatricians. Even though most babies are born without trouble of any kind, an emergency situation can occur at any time, without advance notice, unexpectedly, and with disastrous results if the obstetrician is not right there and the pediatrician easily available. A cord around the neck, a sudden hemorrhage, an infant who is not breathing, a rapid onset of jaundice are all complications common enough to demand attention and serious enough to strike terror into the hearts of anyone not completely surrounded by the protective technology and skilled personnel of the modern hospital.

If a baby is born prematurely, or, more accurately, not weighing enough (less than 5.5 lbs, for example), or if he weighs too much or if his condition is poor for other reasons, or if he is deformed in any way, then his best chance for survival lies in immediate transfer, via special ambulance and trained attendants, to a "high-risk center" where technology and personnel of an even more sophisticated advanced order are available and waiting to take over. Soon these perinatal care centers will be available in every region of our great country so that no one need be without care.

Thus, fetal monitoring and amniocentesis before birth are supplemented by special incubators, oxygen, artificial breathing supports, temperature regulation, intravenous fluids, and monitoring apparatus after birth to give maximum help regardless of the infant's poor condition.

Now, many newborns who get into trouble, despite the best of medical care, do so because of their mothers. It is well known that many mothers in America, especially among the poor, are still too ignorant and stupid to seek out prenatal care; plenty of them smoke, drink, and take pot; others are too lazy and uninterested to shop properly and eat right despite their doctor's advice and the availability of nutritious food (including through government programs for the poor) to everyone. Is it any wonder that they have such a high rate of premature infants, many of whom remain in trouble physically and emotionally their entire lives.

* ROBERT S. MENDELSOHN is Associate Professor, Department of Preventive Medicine, Lincoln School of Medicine, University of Illinois; Author of the nationally syndicated newspaper column, "The People's Doctor"; Vice President, Society for the Protection of the Unborn Thru Nutrition; Medical Advisor, La Leche League International; and Co-Founder of the American College of Home Obstetrics.

WHEN IT COMES TO CARING FOR CHILDREN, ONE GRANDMOTHER
IS WORTH TWO PEDIATRICIANS.

Yet, in spite of these irresponsible, breeding mothers, the
generous and humane impulses of American science guarantee that
everything will be done to help their offspring survive--even though
unwanted in many instances. While some would question whether it is
ethically correct to save these babies, thus adding to the total burden of the world's population, quantitatively and qualitatively,
American doctors are not judgmental, and no sacrifice on their part
is too great to insure a successful infant outcome.

MODERN PEDIATRIC, HIGH-RISK NURSERY CARE, EVEN FOR THE
BABY AT RISK, HAS NOT BEEN PROVEN TO OFFER ANY ADVANTAGE
ABOVE SOME OF THE ALTERNATIVES TO THIS APPROACH.

It is practically impossible to change the behavior of these
women, often referred to as "disadvantaged," as much as we doctors
would dearly love to do so. But, after all, we find it hard to
change the attitudes of even rich and middle-class women who, despite
all of our attempts to influence them, still largely prefer to have
their babies delivered on schedule by induction, want to be knocked
out, don't want their husbands to see them in this shape, and reject
breastfeeding. Given the nature of the American women, all that we
male MD's can do is work within that framework and use all of our
skills and machinery to overcome the damage done either by maternal
habits or acts of God.

I LIKE NURSE MIDWIVES AND THEY MAKE ME COMFORTABLE SO
LONG AS THEY DON'T BEGIN TO ACT LIKE PHYSICIANS.

In the best of all possible worlds, and we expect this to come
within the next few years, we will have neonatologists and regional-
ized perinatal care centers within easy reach of the entire population, and amniocentesis, monitoring, and other specialized services
available to all.

LOOK AT THE LONG LIST OF MEDICAL "ADVANCES" THAT WERE
ALL STATISTICALLY "PROVEN" UNTIL THEY WERE LATER STATIS-
TICALLY DISPROVEN--THUS PASSING FROM THE REALM OF THE CERTAIN INTO
THE REALM OF THE CONTROVERSIAL.

QUESTIONS

So much for a description of *conventional* attitudes, and I can
assure you from my daily contacts with doctors and from reading medical literature that this picture is accurately stated. However, the
important questions are: Is it true? And is it desirable? I would
suggest a number of issues:

1. Are high-risk centers of any value? Do they really decrease mortality, or is this another example of the ever-growing body of self-serving medical statistics. Look at the long list of "advances" that were all statistically proven until they were later statistically disproven, thus passing from the realm of certainty into the realm of the controversial.

2. Do doctors deserve the credit for the fall in infant mortality over the past 70-80 years? Or perhaps, infant mortality was very low centuries ago when midwives delivered babies at home. When the female healer, including the midwife, was eliminated through the witch hunts of the 17th and 18th centuries, male doctors took over. They had one characteristic that midwives did not possess--i.e. they performed autopsies. And they had a nasty habit of going from the autopsy table to the mother in ·labor without washing their hands or, judging from old pictures, without even changing their bloody gowns. Is it any wonder that childbirth fever--puerperal sepsis--became the great killer of these times?

Finally, of course, toward the end of the 19th century, Ignacz Semmelweiss told the doctors "wash your hands, ·you damn fools," for which his final reward was incarceration in an insane asylum. And, as the male doctors began to wash their hands, childbirth fever began to disappear.

Now, my concern is that modern medicine has taken credit for the decline in infant mortality, but understandably enough, has never considered assuming *blame* for its previous rise.

3. Is a modern, highly expensive, fully equipped and staffed infant incubator better, worse, or the same as the simple, inexpensive, old-fashioned incubator that leaked oxygen so badly there was no opportunity to reach levels that would, and did, cause an epidemic of blindness that affected thousands and thousands of babies.

4. How safe are bilirubin lights for jaundice? Are they as safe as thalidomide? DES to mothers? Irradiation of tonsils and other procedures all originally hailed as *safe* by ever-trusting medical researchers? Now there are cases of blood-incompatibility jaundice, though rare, that do require treatment. But the common, normal physiologic type of jaundice is different. There is no good evidence that jaundice is helped by hospitalization. As a matter of fact, there is a lot of evidence that some of the stuff we do for jaundiced babies is plenty dangerous. My general rule, as a pediatrician, with few exceptions, is that if a baby is jaundiced and happens to be in the hospital and it's on the first or second day and the mother says, "What should I do because the obstetrician and the neonatologists are already in to drawing blood and everything else?" my answer is, "Get the baby out of the hospital before anybody else sees the jaundice and go home."

5. Will the high noise levels of incubators cause a new epidemic of deafness?

6. Since the feeding of human milk to high-risk babies is a rare occurrence, what about the incidence of high blood lead levels and sudden infant death (SIDS) characteristic of formula-fed babies?

7. Since the incidence of prematurity (small weight babies) has not decreased, and there is some evidence that it is increasing, perhaps the emphasis on treatment after the fact has obscured the opportunities to prevent babies from becoming "high risk." We already know how to prevent prematurity; but why should the "high-risk" industry work itself out of business? After all, without prematurity how would 90% of all neonatologists make a living?

8. The modern management of high-risk mothers and infants has led to an epidemic of learning disorders, emotional disturbance, and mental retardation in later life. Physicians claim that this is the price of success, or as one said, "our failures result from our success." I question this self-serving puffery that assumes that decreasing mortality results in increasing morbidity. In the first place, U.S. mortality is still quite high in comparison with other countries. Furthermore, the survival rate for small infants (20%-23% die) has remained practically unchanged since the 1920s (except as modified by some tricky statisticians). I would argue that both mortality and morbidity travel in the *same* direction and are *not* reciprocal. Therefore, the "advantage" of modern treatment remains in the realm of speculation--particularly as the risks and the dangers become more obvious.

My presentation deals with "Childbirth Alternatives and Infant Outcome." In one sentence, my contention is that modern pediatric, high-risk nursery care, even for the baby at risk, has not been proven to offer any advantage to well conceived alternatives such as would be afforded by the home environment. So if anybody says to you that "home delivery is dangerous," the answer is that "as far as we know at this point, hospital delivery for normals is dangerous and, as far as we know, for at-risk babies hospitals may be even more dangerous."

I view a hospital like war. You try not to get into it, but if you have to get in, you try to get out as soon as you can.

You who are starting out by having babies at home are not only helping your baby to a healthier life and decreasing his chances of minimal brain damage, learning disabilities, and everything else, but you are also helping yourself, your husband, the grandparents, the aunts, the cousins, and everybody else in the family. We have to remember that the kind of family we are interested in is not the kind you learned about in the Primer where they have father, mother, Dick, Jane, and Spot. We are interested in the *entire* family and the wonderful thing about homebirth is that everybody can be in on the game.

Just to show you how families can be separated in one hospital with which I am connected, they allow *one* visitor at every visiting period and the mother has to choose between her mother, her mother-in-law, and her husband. I don't know of a better way to break up families.

In summary, then, let me say that I think that if you take a look at the complications that everybody is worried about today as far as the newborn is concerned, you would have to question whether the hospital is the optimal place in which to deal with them.

PREDICTIONS

Crystal-ball gazing is always chancy, but lots of fun; and furthermore, since I am committing myself to writing, you will be able to judge my ability as a seer in years to come and decide on that basis whether to include me among those invited to future meetings. So here are my predictions:

1. The perinatal center movement will continue to expand for several more years, costing the country millions of dollars.

2. During this time, as has happened in many other fields of medicine, the negative scientific and statistical studies on high-risk centers will emerge, leading to widespread justified skepticism on the part of both professionals and the public. At the same time, scientific studies of better methods will become available. I am introducing, along with my presentation here (see p. 37), a splendid example of this kind of study, one entitled, "Comparative Study of Obstetrics," by Frederic M. Ettner, MD, wherein the risks and disadvantages of normal hospital-based obstetrical practice are described and documented, citing over 50 references, and compared to the statistics of a home birth sample from a physicians' "Home Obstetrics" service in Chicago. Even though Dr. Ettner is a very young man, I believe this is a landmark document in the world of medical science and deserves the widest possible distribution. I urge you to pay close attention, not only to Dr. Ettner's data, but also to the highly effective rhetorical phrases he has collected, including:

* "just in case" medicine
* "the extreme becomes the rule"
* "iatrogenocide"
* "medical mastectomy"
* "shoveling the sidewalk before the snow falls"

3. NAPSAC and like-minded organizations will build up a solid base of professional and public support with skillful use of the communications media.

4. Public disillusionment with the high cost and poor yield of modern prenatal, natal, and neonatal care will express itself politically in demands for abolition of high-risk nurseries (recognized as being of high risk for the babies) and replacement with true methods of prevention.

5. Tom Brewer will be recognized as the Ignacz Semmelweiss of the 20th century and his vigorous teaching and leadership will make obsolete modern prenatal and perinatal care. Tom's happy outlook on life will, however, insure his avoiding Semmelweiss' fate.

6. Doris Haire will write a sequel to her present best-selling publication, probably named "The Cultural Warping of Modern Pediatrics."

7. Establishment medicine dies hard, and it will probably require a series of legal actions, including malpractice suits against individual physicians, to bring the lesson home to the great majority of doctors. People like me and organizations like NAPSAC will be asked to give testimony and otherwise participate in securing patients' legal rights to compensation for damage being done which is known to be preventable right now.

8. As (1) maternal nutrition improves, (2) home deliveries increase, (3) elective induction, episiotomies, and anesthesia-anal-gesia disappear--high-risk pregnancies will all but vanish. Neona-tologists will have to seek honest employment and most high-risk centers will become museums.

9. Home-based obstetrics will be recognized as a separate specialty, for which the average hospital-based obstetrician is not qualified by either training, temperament, or experience.

10. NAPSAC will shorten its name, since there is really no safe alternative to our (AOHO) teaching.

11. There will be a more organized, structured relationship of NAPSAC and all organizations working against the present irrational system.

12. Many families, including our own, will have saved their infants from our present risky hospital deliveries.

13. This May 15, 1976, meeting will be regarded as an historic event--probably the best happening of the Bicentennial Year.

If our government ever really wants to set up a good department they should set up a Department of Doctor Produced Diseases (DDPD) and begin to disseminate real information like the kind presented at this conference because there are two things we have to do: (1) We have to build things up, and there's plenty of building up, construc-tive effort going on, and (2) at the same time we have to tear down. In order to learn anything new, you have got to learn everything that was wrong before. That's why I am in favor of a combined destructive-constructive approach simultaneously.

Today we are in the midst of a political campaign in this country and we are asking all kinds of questions of the candidates. Maybe we are asking the wrong set of questions. I think I'd like to know whether they were born in a hospital or at home? I'd like to know if their mothers were sedated? Did they have pink toes or blue toes? I want to know how long it took them to breathe? I want to know if they were breastfed or bottle fed? I want to know what they and their wives are doing with their own children. Because there *is* a difference in the outcomes of in and out-of-hospital birth exper-iences, these may be the most important questions in determining the intelligence and capability of a Presidential Candidate.

In conclusion, let me thank you very much for giving this pediatrician the opportunity to contrast infant outcome of present-day modern medicine with that of the NAPSAC-inspired future. Lucky for us here today, the future is now. I am happy to share it with you.

Comparative Study of Obstetrics
With Data & Details of a Working Physician's Home OB Service

Frederic M. Ettner, MD, ACHO*

Conventional hospital obstetric practices in the United States have been founded, shaped, and influenced largely by cultural, economic and commercial pressures. Many of our accepted practices are not supported by scientific research and appear to be rooted more in hospital and medical professional tradition than in human physiology. Dr. Roberto Caldeyro-Barcia, an expert on the problems of birth for the World Health Organization and President-elect of the International Federation of Gynecologists and Obstetricians has stated that several common American obstetrical practices used in labor and delivery were potentially dangerous to the health of the baby about to be born.[1] Both Doris Haire, former President of the International Childbirth Education Association, and photo-journalist, Suzanne Arms, have described women and childbirth in America precisely via the titles of their respective publications: "The Cultural Warping of Childbirth" and "Immaculate Deception."

However, no study has evaluated or described childbirth at home from the standpoint of clinical obstetrical data and anecdotal case study in a varied urban population as compared to the present mode of normal hospital obstetrics. Through observation and participation in the home delivery process, this present report describes home delivery as a *superior* method of handling normal obstetrics. The disadvantages and risks of normal hospital-based obstetrical practice will be described with documentation cited.

Our original intent was to compare this home delivery method with that of a similarly selected urban population possessing similar characteristics in a hospital setting. However, a careful search of the literature and personal interviews with authorities in the fields of Obstetrics-Gynecology (Dr. Michael Newton, Professor of Obstetrics-Gynecology at the University of Chicago Pritzker School of Medicine and former Executive Director, American College of Obstetrics & Gynecology) and Preventive Medicine-Community Health (Dr. Edward Lichter, Chairman of the Department of Preventive Medicine and Community Health at the University of Illinois, Abraham Lincoln School of Medicine) reveals an absence of studies in this specific clinical setting. This paper will provide an introduction for future studies involving private hospital-based obstetrics and home deliveries in the cities of San Francisco, Green Bay, and Chicago. The present study can provide a standard against which future comparisons can be made, at which time statistical analysis will be feasible.

---

* *FREDERIC M. ETTNER is presently at the Cook County Hospital in Chicago and has received training in an Urban Preceptorship Program in home-based obstetrics under the guidelines of the American College of Home Obstetrics and is a Charter Member of the American College of Home Obstetrics.*

CONVENTIONAL OBSTETRICS - 1975

Although the stated objective of the health sciences today is to promote full normal human development, it is apparent that hospital obstetrical practice in the U.S. has affected something grossly less than the above ideal. In an attempt to manage the 4%-7% of pathologic obstetrics[2], with the full support of scientific research and a panoply of drugs, the treatment of exceptional cases has become the rule. Not only has the normal pregnant woman been subjected to the rigors of prophylactic obstetrical care during delivery, but also pre- and postnatally. This method of obstetrical prophylaxis has been described by Suzanne Arms as "just-in-case" obstetrical science. The image is an attending obstetrician intervening only when labor deviates from normal; the reality is preventive intervention for *all* pregnant women. The reality of the "exceptions becoming the rule" is exemplified on obstetrical wards throughout the entire country.

IN AN ATTEMPT TO MANAGE THE 4-7% OF TRULY PATHOLOGIC OBSTETRICS, THE TREATMENT FOR EXCEPTIONAL CASES HAS BECOME THE RULE. THIS HAS BEEN DESCRIBED BY SUZANNE ARMS AS "JUST-IN-CASE" OBSTETRICS.

This kind of preventive medicine has been referred to by the apocryphal phrase, "shoveling the sidewalk before the snow falls."[3] The following are examples of this kind of medical practice:

* The exception: an obese, symptomatic pregnant woman who is in need of close scrutiny concerning nutrition and weight gain; the rule: surveillance of all pregnant women with respect to added pounds and enforcing limits, diets, and medications.

* The exception: a long, tiring pre-labor which may require sedation; the rule: sedation for almost all delivering mothers.

* The exception: an intravenous pathway to administer anesthesia and/or analgesia and physiologic fluids for emergency surgical intervention; the rule: routine intravenous fluids in order to keep a vein open for the remote possibility of a surgical procedure.

* The exception: surgical intervention, i.e., Caesarean section, prohibiting liquids or food by mouth; the rule: non pars oris for all.

* The exception: a poorly contracting uterus unable to expel its contents requiring synthetic oxytocin; the rule: oxytocin routinely to prevent hemorrhage and aid in expelling the placenta.

* The exception: vaginal incompetence requiring episiotomy; the rule: prophylactic episiotomies prior to delivery of the baby's head for most mothers.

* The exception: use of low forceps in arrested mid-late second stage labor; the rule: use of forceps in all deliveries.

* The exception: confinement to a hospital bed for the infrequent cases of cardiac and respiratory compromised women; the rule: hospital bed confinement for all.

The pediatrician joins the obstetrician in this perverted scheme. Thus, the exception: encouragement to breastfeed; the rule: universal formula feeding via bottle; the hazard: resultant damage to a healthy baby. (A summary of the above is presented in Table 1 on the following page)

The result of all these practices is a scientific systematic protocol of preventive interferences perverting normals into abnormals and, thereby, deviating from the natural process. All of the preceding statements make it advisable, indeed, mandatory, to re-evaluate these common medical practices. However, these attitudes have become traditional, time-honored concepts handed down uncritically by the overwhelming majority of physicians. There exists an almost blanket refusal by the Medical Establishment to investigate the ramifications of their prophylactic, "just-in-case" obstetrical science.

THE SIGNIFICANCE OF BIRTH WEIGHT

The weight of an infant at birth is an important developmental milestone. In conjunction with gestational age, it provides a useful index of intrauterine growth. Intrauterine growth not only reflects the developmental experience of the fetus, but also predicts fetal outcome--both immediate and long range.[4] If one considers birth weight with respect to perinatal outcome, there exists overwhelming evidence that if a large amount of information currently available about factors that influence birth weight were fully utilized, medically and socially, the frequency of low birth weight could appreciably be reduced and thereby lower perinatal morbidity and mortality.[5] The relationship between low birth weight (i.e. 2500 grams or 5.5 lbs and below, formerly designated as prematurity) and increased risk of adverse outcome is well known. This fact was documented by Dr. W.J. Little as far back as 1862 when he linked low birth weight and cerebral palsy. Because low birth weight is a common condition, the problem of physical and intellectual impairment is one of large dimension.[6] Dr. Tom Brewer of Contra Costa, California, and formerly of the University of California, San Francisco, has repeatedly stated with extensive documentation the consequences of malnutrition in human pregnancy--specifically that of protein starvation and metabolic toxemia of late pregnancy. If one were to list factors affecting birth weight, the strongest correlation exists between the amount of weight gained by the mother during pregnancy and her pre-pregnant state, with the weight of the infant at birth.[7]

Brewer states that one out of every ten newborn infants has low birth weight, and increasing numbers of defective children are being born to women in all economic classes. These physically and neurologically deformed children are often the result of poor nutrition of the mothers.[8] In Brewer's book, "Metabolic Toxemia of Late Pregnancy," he substantiates his claim with personal research and an extensive bibliography. Brewer attacks the common obstetrical practice of arbitrarily limiting the weight gain of a pregnant woman, which often results in administration of diuretics and a salt-free diet. Not only will this regimen continue to threaten our nation with an epidemic of low-weight, premature, mentally retarded or physically deformed children, but via this practice the maternal disease of metabolic toxemia is actually increased.[9]

TABLE 1

EXAMPLES OF ROUTINE PRACTICE OF PROCEDURES ORIGINALLY ONLY INTENDED FOR THE EXCEPTION

EXCEPTION	RULE	HAZARD
1. Careful attention to weight of grossly obese, symptomatic women	Tight weight restrictions for all	Increased incidence of toxemia and prematurity
2. Prolonged pre-labor requiring sedation	Sedation for almost all laboring mothers	Potentially narcotized infant with possible severe respiratory and neurologic complications
3. Intravenous pathway to administer anesthesia for the possibility of surgical intervention	IV's for all	Narcotized infant with potentially severe respiratory and neurologic complications; IV fluid contamination
4. Artificial rupture of membranes to shorten prolonged second stage of labor	Premature artificial rupture of membranes during early labor routinely	Cephalic compression, cranial hypertension, cerebral birth trauma (and neurological sequelae)
5. Administering of synthetic oxytocin for elective induction; or to stimulate an atonic uterus	Synthetic oxytocin to initiate or facilitate uniform uterine contractions for most	Cephalic compression, cranial hypertension, cerebral birth trauma (and neurological sequelae); episodes of cerebral ischemia with permanent CNS depression
6. Vaginal incompetence requiring episiotomy	Routine prophylactic episiotomies	Increased perinatal infection & trauma; increased blood loss; fetal complications of local anesthesia
7. Low forceps in arrested mid-late 2nd stage after infusion of synthetic hormones, anesthesia and/or analgesia	Use of forceps in almost all deliveries	Fetal cephalic injury with subsequent neurologic sequelae; iatrogenic skeletal dislocations and subluxations.
8. Confinement to hospital bed during pre-labor and 1st stage for cardiac and respiratory compromised women	Confinement to hospital bed during pre-labor and 1st stage for all women	Compromised uterine circulation, postural hypotension, muscle weakness, less effective uterine contractions

The etiology of metabolic toxemia of late pregnancy was observed and documented forty years ago by Dr. M.B. Strauss[10] & Dr. R.A. Ross[11]. However, it is apparent that aside from Dr. Brewer, not one obstetrician has *publically and vigorously* condemned these time-honored concepts and practices of limiting weight gain, salt-free diets and medications to enhance rapid loss of weight in pregnant women. If the answers to these problems include adequate protein intake and a weight gain of *at least 25 pounds* by the mother, as proven by Strauss[12] and Brewer[13], a reduction in the incidence of toxemia will be observed with concomitant improved neonatal survival. In the Collaborative Perinatal Study of the National Institute of Neurological Diseases and Stroke the data indicate that a maternal weight gain of *25 pounds and greater* yielded the lowest rates of perinatal mortality and delivery of low birth weight infants.[14]

However, the question remains: "Why does iatrogenic starvation of pregnant women continue with the ensuing complications of increased rate of prematurity and metabolic toxemia of late pregnancy?" Brewer argues that no country can call itself "developed" as long as even one of its citizens, least of all a pregnant woman, is deprived of an adequate protein and caloric intake and allowed to go hungry.[15]

DRUGS IN PREGNANCY AND BIRTH

Brewer's other theses include: that there is practically no place for medication in pregnancy; that low salt diets are dangerous, as are diuretics; that stress on weight loss or gain is irrelevant; and, emphatically, that good plentiful sound nutrition is the main foundation for a healthy mother and baby.

Drugs utilized by pregnant women, either prescribed by a physician or taken over-the-counter, can have both determined and undetermined adverse affects on pre and postnatal development. Despite accelerated research in developmental pharmacology and improved surveillance procedures prompted by the thalidomide episode, very little additional information has been forthcoming concerning the extent to which drugs contribute to impaired physical and mental development in the human being, or concerning the precise mechanism by which they exert their adverse affects.[16] Yet drugs continue to be prescribed without warning to pregnant women in all stages of gestation. Unsuspecting women, newborns, and children are the grim reapers of these continued practices, which reach their zenith in the hospital.

THERE IS PRACTICALLY NO PLACE FOR MEDICATION IN PREGNANCY; LOW SALT DIETS ARE DANGEROUS, AS ARE DIURETICS; STRESS ON WEIGHT LOSS OR GAIN IS IRRELEVANT; AND GOOD PLENTIFUL SOUND NUTRITION IS THE MAIN FOUNDATION FOR A HEALTHY MOTHER AND BABY.

THOMAS H. BREWER, MD

In a report of the Committee on Maternal Health, the American College of Obstetricians and Gynecologists in 1970, with Dr. Michael Newton as Executive Director, surveyed 80% of the hospital births in the United States. This extensive compilation revealed that: 82% of the hospitals reported that *almost all* (80-100%) of their patients

received obstetric analgesia; 81% of the hospitals reported that
almost all (80-100%) of their patients received obstetric anesthesia;
inhalation anesthesia was the most frequently used anesthesia for
vaginal deliveries.[17]

Virtually all drugs administered during pregnancy pass the placental barrier to a greater or lesser degree and, thus, are at least
a potential threat to the fetus.[18] A more precise definition of placental function in transport of electrolytes, metabolites, and drugs
would label it a sieve, not a barrier.

Drugs ingested by the mother may affect the fetus indirectly
either by initiating metabolic changes in the mother or exerting a
physiologic effect on the placenta adverse to the fetus. During the
very early stages of pregnancy, that of rapid cellular proliferation,
drugs may cause abortion or induce chromosomal aberrations. Since
many women are unaware of their pregnancy, these embryo-toxic effects
may go unrecognized. Developmental defects can be induced via drug
administration during organogenesis in the fetus. Externally visible
malformations may be recognized at birth, but internal malformations
such as cardiac or renal anomalies or mental retardation may not be
apparent for years after birth when an association with drug intake
might be hard to establish.[19]

ASPHYXIA NEONATORUM, BRADYCARDIA, LOWERED PH, NEUROLOGICAL
INJURY, SEIZURES, TWITCHING, OPISTHOTONOS, INCESSANT CRYING,
DEPRESSION, FLACCIDITY, AGITATION-HYPERIRRITABILITY, AND DEATH IN
THE NEWBORN PERIOD, AMONG OTHERS, ARE SOME OF THE APPARENT ADVERSE
EFFECTS OF PARACERVICAL ANESTHESIA.

The common practice of administering analgesia and/or anesthesia
in term pregnancy during labor can result in toxic manifestations for
the neonate, particularly the premature infant. In the tradition of
obstetrical science, pain in the laboring woman has evoked many therapeutic approaches. However, the safety of local anesthetics in routine vaginal deliveries and subsequent effects on the neonate have
been seriously questioned, and doubt raised concerning this so-called
therapeutic regimen. There is evidence that local anesthetics administered by epidural, caudal, or paracervical routes rapidly reach
fetal and maternal circulation in measurable concentrations.[20] Extensive documentation reveals that the technique of administering the
anesthetic via injection may inadvertently reach the fetus *itself*,
and that effects of paracervical anesthesia will remain for a protracted period of time since detoxification by the newborn's liver is
slow.[21] The effects of local anesthetics, which reach almost all newborns,[17] range from depression to neurological sequelae and infant
death. Asphyxia neonatorum, bradycardia, lowered pH, neurological
injury, i.e., seizures, twitching, opisthotonos, incessant crying,
depression, flaccidity,   agitation-hyperirritability, and death in
the newborn period, among others, are some of the apparent adverse
affects of *paracervical* anesthesia.[20,22,23] Although thoughtful re-
consideration of the administration of local anesthetics is warrented
by the obstetrician, this common practice remains unabated. Dr. Guillozet summarizes by asking, "Is the immature nervous system of the

fetus being assaulted and are the true risks of local anesthetic agents unassessed, unrevealed, and perhaps unwarranted in the uncomplicated vaginal delivery?"[21]

In 1958 the virilizing effect of progestins and other hormone preparations on the fetus in the treatment of threatened abortion was first reported. It is now well documented in studies by Greenwald et al.[24] and Barner et al.[25] that vaginal adenosis and adenocarcinoma occur in adolescent girls and young women whose mothers received diethylstilbestrol (DES) during pregnancy for threatened abortion.

---

80 % OF CONGENITAL ANOMALIES CAN BE ATTRIBUTED TO RAMPANT ADMINISTRATION OF DRUGS AND EVEN A HIGHER PERCENTAGE OF DEFECTS IN STILLBIRTHS AND ABORTIONS CAN BE ATTRIBUTED TO DRUGS.

F.O. KELSEY, MD

Thalidomide produced profound effects on the developing fetus in very low dosages, whereas it exhibited little or no apparent adverse effects in the mother even with dosages well above the therapeutic range. Defects including deafness, blindness, limb deformities, cardiac, renal, and intestinal anomalies were observed. Investigations conducted even after the thalidomide episode indicate that on the average between three and four drugs are prescribed during pregnancy.[16] Dr. F.O. Kelsey, Director of the scientific investigation staff for the Bureau of Drug and Food Administration, attributes the unknown etiology of 80% of congenital anomalies to rampant administration of drugs. A higher percentage of defects in stillbirths and abortions can be attributed to drugs. The possibilities and permutations of drug combinations and interactions with genetic factors and environmental chemicals (i.e. pesticides and food additives) are reaching frightening proportions.[16]

NURSES AND WOMEN ANESTHESIOLOGISTS WORKING IN OPERATING ROOMS EXPERIENCE A GREATER RATE OF SPONTANEOUS ABORTION THAN THE POPULATION IN GENERAL.

Kelsey cites the teratogenic manifestations of anticonvulsants, i.e., diphenylhydantoin, trimethadione, and paramethadione. Diphenylhydantoin not only is transported, via the placenta to the fetus, but serum samples have indicated higher concentrations of the drug in fetal blood than that in maternal blood. Anomalies including cleft lip and/or palate have been observed in their offspring. Ingestion of trimethadione and paramethadione in epileptic mothers has been associated with a variety of congenital malformations including mild mental retardation.[16]

The adverse effects of anesthesia are not limited to the delivering mother and newborn. Reports from Norway and the United States indicate that nurses and women anesthesiologists working in operating rooms experience a greater rate of spontaneous abortion than the population in general.[16]

Many other drugs have been implicated in causing congenital malformations. Aspirin, probably the most common and most readily available drug, has a high association with congenital defects. Mothers receiving opiates therapeutically during pregnancy for diarrhea, and as analgesia during labor, deliver narcotized neonates who experience withdrawal symptoms. Over-the-counter cough remedies include iodides which may lead to goiter formation in the fetus that may be sufficiently extensive to depress respirations or interfere with delivery. Treatment of a hyperthyroid woman not known to be pregnant with radioiodine can result in cretinism in her offspring.[16] Sulfonamides, the antibiotic novobiocin, nitrofurans and water-soluble vitamin K analogs, all drugs commonly prescribed to mothers in their third trimester, will precipitate jaundice in the newborn (i.e. displacement of bilirubin bound to albumin and/or hemolytic effect on immature red blood cells).[16,26]

ASPIRIN HAS A HIGH ASSOCIATION WITH CONGENITAL DEFECTS.

Dr. Tom Brewer has vigorously campaigned against the use of drugs in pregnancy, especially diuretics, yet they continue to be prescribed on a large scale by obstetricians. The prestigious medical journals, "Obstetrics and Gynecology" and "The American Journal of Obstetrics and Gynecology" are filled with advertisements enticing the willing, unquestioning clinician to prescribe their magic potions. Although the documentation is precise and the warnings of mutagenic effects, the development of cancer, mental and/or behavioral aberrations affecting the central nervous system in the fetus and newborn are distinct-- yet the prescribing physician remains steadfast on a course of "iatrogenocide."[42]

ELECTIVE INDUCTION

In a one day meeting in New York City, April 9, 1975, of the American Foundation for Maternal and Child Health, Dr. Roberto Caldeyro-Barcia issued grave warnings concerning the common obstetrical practices in the United States. These practices include the elective induction and stimulation of labor with drugs, and/or artificially rupturing the amniotic membranes early in labor, and keeping the woman lying on her back during labor and delivery.

The elective induction of labor via synthetic oxytocin has become common practice in obstetrics. In Great Britain the point has now been reached in some units that half or more of all patients are *not* permitted to go into spontaneous labor.[27] Dr. Caldeyro-Barcia notes that elective induction rates in private hospitals in the United States are up to 35% of all deliveries. Latin American statistics reveal a lower incidence of elective induction in public maternities, but in private practice the incidence is similar to that found in the United States.[28] The ultimate consequence of this time-honored practice is painfully clear: *one perinatal death in 200 elective inductions of labor.*[29,30] Statistics gathered by the National Institutes of Health indicate that labor, in at least 1 in 5 births in this country, is stimulated by oxytocin. Additionally, in at least 1 in 10 births, labor is actually induced by drugs. The numbers affected amount to about one million American babies each year.

The hormone oxytocin is naturally secreted by the posterior pituitary and stimulates uterine contractions, and in a term pregnancy the uterus will expel its contents--the baby and placenta. However, even when synthetic oxytocin is given at physiological doses under strict control, it is impossible to reproduce exactly the pattern of spontaneous contractility of labor. Dr. Caldeyro-Barcia has demonstrated that uterine contractions stimulated with synthetic oxytocin reach over 40 mm Hg pressure on the fetal head. Needless to say, the intensity of contractions was significantly higher in induced labors than in spontaneous labors.[27]

Even under optimal conditions, in so-called "favorable obstetric conditions," involving scheduled term pregnancies, inductions are not favorable for the fetus. The quality and quantity of uterine contractions are greatly affected in oxytocin enhanced labor. The contractions tend to be stronger, longer, and with shorter relaxation periods between. As a result, the fetus is compromised before its first breath. The rapidity and strength of contractions decrease the ability of the fetus to restore its supply of oxygen. With each uterine contraction, blood supply to the uterus is temporarily shut off.   If deprived of blood supply, a fetal bradycardia follows with oxygen deprivation and cerebral ischemia causing the grave possibility of neurological sequelae.[31]

EVEN UNDER THE MOST FAVORABLE OBSTETRIC CONDITIONS,
INDUCTION IS NOT FAVORABLE FOR THE FETUS.

Induction of labor is indicated in specified clinical settings, those cases in which continuation of pregnancy would present an absolute threat to the life or well being of the mother or her child: examples include severe pre-eclampsia, severe uncontrolled diabetes mellitus, severe Rh sensitization, previous history of severe hemorrhage, and greatly prolonged pregnancy. If these practices were performed only when indicated, *at most, 3% of births* would be affected, according to Dr. Caldeyro-Barcia. The rate of indiscriminate induction is exemplified by the following: in the month of May, 1975, at a private medical-school-affiliated hospital in Metropolitan Chicago 55% of all deliveries were induced with synthetic oxytocin. It is obvious that the indications for induction have become much broader and therefore inclusive of: (1) the social convenience of the mother or her obstetrician, (2) the medical convenience of a daylight delivery when expert staff are available and at the peak of their efficiency, and (3) electively induced deliveries "at term" in which an error in calculating a due date may result in a premature child with irreparable damage.[27] These broader indications reveal a trend of meddlesome midwifery interfering with a delicately balanced natural process. Unfortunately, the risks are to the unborn child alone, without an avenue of complaint. In summary, *most* cases of neonatal damage are mainly due to the iatrogenic prematurity caused by the elective induction.[31]

MOST CASES OF NEONATAL DAMAGE ARE DUE TO IATROGENIC
PREMATURITY CAUSED BY ELECTIVE INDUCTION.

IF INDUCTION WERE PERFORMED ONLY WHEN TRULY MEDICALLY
INDICATED, AT MOST, ONLY 3 % OF BIRTHS WOULD BE AFFECTED;
YET, THE RATE OF INDISCRIMINANT INDUCTION IS OVER 50 % IN SOME
AMERICAN HOSPITALS.

Stimulation of labor is indicated when uterine contractions
are too weak and/or infrequent, arresting the normal progression of
the neonate through the birth canal. Artificial rupture of amniotic
membranes or the administration of synthetic oxytocin stimulates an
arrested labor. Evidence from the extensive obstetrical clinical
observations by Drs. R.L. Schwarcz, R. Caldeyro-Barcia, and associates concerning the fetus and early rupture of the membranes reveals conclusive facts in conflict with this common obstetrical practice in the management of labor.[33]

ARTIFICIAL RUPTURE OF MEMBRANES

The membranes contain amniotic fluid serving as a protective
balloon encompassing the fetus. When the membranes are intact, pressure received at any single point on the fetus is equally distributed
especially around the fetal head (Pascal's Law).[33] Since the membranes are intact, counterpressure will be exerted via amniotic fluid
preventing excessive misalignment and/or deformity of the bones comprising the fetal head. Not only is uterine contractile pressure
equalized on the fetal head but also on the fetal body, umbilical
cord and placenta.[32] It is important to note that uterine contractions with intact membranes produce no changes in blood flow through
the fetal brain.[32]

Schwarcz and Caldeyro-Barcia have gathered extensive physiologic data on the pressure exerted by uterine contractions on the head
of the human fetus during labor. During advanced labor proximal to
delivery of the fetus, following the natural rupture of the membranes
each uterine contraction may cause a transient fall in the fetal
heart rate. It has been postulated that each transient fall in the
fetal heart rate is caused by a strong compression exerted on the
fetal head by the corresponding uterine contraction. The noted
decrease in fetal heart rate is effected by cephalic compression
mediated via the vagus nerve. This normal physiologic periodicity of
the fetal heart rate due to uterine contractions is of no consequence
except when rupture of membranes is artificially effected early in
the first stage of labor.[32, 33]

AS PUBLIC AWARENESS INCREASES CONCERNING THE DANGERS AND
RISKS OF CONVENTIONAL HOSPITAL-BASED OBSTETRICS, WILL
THESE COMMON DELIVERY TECHNIQUES IMPOSE LEGAL HAZARDS TO
PHYSICIANS LEADING TO MALPRACTICE CHARGES? THERE ARE SAFER
ALTERNATIVES.

With the early artificial rupture of membranes the fetal head
is defenseless through the tortuous course of the pelvis and birth
canal. If counterpressure via membranes containing a buffeting solution of fluid is eliminated early in labor, the bulging of the unsu-
tured bones in the fetal head is facilitated with concomitant scalp
hemorrhages. The rise of intracranial pressure will be higher than
that in amniotic pressure, with a consequent reduction in cranial
blood flow. Significant decreases in the fetal heart rate via vagal
stimulation is associated with uneven compression and deformation of
the fetal head causing potential cerebral trauma and neurological
defects. Since the bones of the fetal head are not fused, some
molding occurs in deliveries; however, if the natural protection
surrounding the fetal skull is eliminated, production of cranial
hypertension initiating cerebral ischemia ensues. One can logically
deduce that a repetition of successive episodes of cerebral ischemia
precipitates deformation of the brain leading to permanent damage of
the central nervous system of the newborn.[31,33] Dr. Roberto Caldeyro-
Barcia implicates American obstetricians as participants in this
common practice; he issues cautious warnings and advises introspec-
tive thought before deciding to rupture membranes.[1,28,31,33]

THE FLAT-ON-THE-BACK POSITION FOR LABOR IS INHERENTLY
HARMFUL FOR EVERY WOMAN AND CHILD--ADVERSELY AFFECTING
PAIN, COMFORT, UTERINE ACTIVITY, AND THE MAINTENANCE OF NORMAL
BLOOD PRESSURE WHILE, AT THE SAME TIME, IT IS THE SEED AND
GENESIS OF ALL THE IATROGENICALLY INDUCED ADVERSE SEQUELAE.

Cellular growth and development of the fetus depends on the
maintenance of normal fetal homeostasis. Fetal homeostasis is de-
pendent on metabolic exchanges with the mother via the placenta. Any
alteration or deviation from the normal exchange process can cause a
reduction in the supply of anabolites to the fetus and a retention
of the catabolites, with consequences such as acidosis. A variety
of factors previously identified may contribute to insufficient fetomaternal exchanges. Uterine contractions augmented by synthetic
oxytocin and/or rupture of membranes are the most important cause in
reducing blood flow to the intervillous space of the placenta.[33]
Other contributing factors initiated by the obstetrician add to the
effects of induced and/or stimulated contractions either by acting
through different physiologic pathways, by potentiating each other
or synergistically culminating in fetal and/or maternal distress.
Factors including intravenous pathways for administering physiologic
electrolyte solutions as potential vehicles for analgesia, anesthesia and/or oxytocin; subsequent deprivation of sufficient carbohydrate to the mother thereby precipitating acidosis; potential arrest
of labor due to analgesics and/or anesthetics necessitating extraction of the uterine contents via forceps and episiotomy--none of
these could be accomplished in an efficient manner without another
factor--*a supine laboring woman*, i.e., lithotomy position.

THE SUPINE POSITION

Barcia[1,34,35] and Adamson et al.[36] and Bienarz et al.[37] have determined that the lithotomy position is the worst position for labor and delivery, adversely affecting pain and comfort, uterine activity, and the maintenance of normal blood pressure.   Not only does the lithotomy position contain intrinsic adverse sequelae, but it is the seed and genesis of all the iatrogenically augmented procedures.

The supine or lithotomy position has become the standard in American obstetrics[35] and without it the obstetrician could not efficiently effect other identified prophylactic interferences.   However, the influence of position during labor and delivery has received scarce attention from clinicians and investigators.   Dr. Caldeyro-Barcia and others have determined that uterine activity is influenced by the position of the mother.   The characteristics and quality of the contractions are weak, irregular, and *frequent* when the laboring woman is supine, but contractions are stronger, more regular and *less* frequent when the woman is on her side, sitting, standing, or squatting.[34,35]

Supine hypotensive syndrome has been described by Caldeyro-Barcia as a drop in diastolic blood pressure due to restrictive lithotomy position in the laboring woman.   He noted that blood pressure values returned to normal with a change from supine to lateral position.   During labor in the supine position, the pressure exerted by the uterus on the abdominal aorta iliac vessels and inferior vena cava is occlusive, depriving blood supply to the uterus and ultimately the supply of oxygen to the fetus.[31,34,35]   Barcia emphasizes that with or without drugs or the occurrence of supine hypotension, the flat-on-the-back position of giving birth is inherently harmful for every woman and child.[38]   He states "except for being hanged by the feet, the supine position is the worst conceivable position for labor and delivery."[1,31,34,35]

The "warping of childbirth" in America begins with a laboring woman flat on her back, according to Doris Haire.   She summarizes the extensive documentation on obstetrical interferences and prophylaxis initiated by the lithotomy position which tends to:

1. Adversely affect the mother's blood pressure, cardiac return and pulmonary ventilation.
2. Decrease the normal intensity of contractions.
3. Inhibit the mother's voluntary efforts to push her baby out spontaneously.
4. Increase the need for forceps and increase the traction necessary for forceps extraction.
5. Inhibit the spontaneous expulsion of the placenta which, in turn, increases the need for cord traction, forced expression or manual removal of the placenta-- procedures which significantly increase the incidence of fetomaternal hemorrhage.
6. Increase the need for episiotomy because of the increased tension on the pelvic floor and the stretching of the perineal tissue. Normal separation of the feet for natural expulsion is about 15-16 inches which is far less than is allowed by the average American delivery table stirrups.[39]

The natural laws and phenomenon of gravity were mathematically
stated by Sir Isaac Newton in the 17th century. American obstetricians have justified the need of clinical interferences by ignoring a
rudiment of nature--Gravity. Without intervention in a normally progressing labor, the standing position and ambulation permit the pelvic inlet to increase when the legs are extended and facilitate entry
of the fetal head into the pelvis via gravity. Squatting is the best
position for actual birth since the diameter of the pelvic outlet
increases by 1.5 centimeters when the legs are flexed and with the
gravitational forces, the baby is delivered.[34,35]

HAZARDS OF ROUTINE IV'S

Another collaborator in the initiation of obstetric intervention
is the intravenous pathway--the insertion of an IV . As a substitute
for light eating, for periods of up to 24 hours or longer, the physio-
logic-like fluids only add to the pathologic environment of an American hospital birth. This avenue of intravenous transport not only
provides a route for the "just-in-case" anesthesia, analgesia and/or
synthetic oxytocin, but also eliminates the need of food and liquid
by mouth. Non pars oris leading to carbohydrate deprivation has been
implicated in the precipitation of metabolic acidosis of the mother,
occurring in approximately 20% of all women in labor and delivery.
The consequences are experienced initially by the fetuses of mothers
with metabolic acidosis and they are more prone to become acidotic
during the course of labor. The lack of fetal distress signs immediately after delivery does not reflect this insult, as infants may
not be depressed at birth.[36] Adamson et al. have described a multi-
tude of events contributing to fetal asphyxia; among these is metabolic acidosis of the mother. He and his associates have proposed
that intrapartum acidosis and hypercarbia are not an inevitable consequence of normal labor, and that under normal unmedicated infusion-
less conditions the fetal acid-base state remains essentially unchanged.
They stress that the supine position and/or anesthesia and/or analgesia imposed upon the laboring patient may have adverse effects upon
placental perfusion, particularly when the autonomic nervous system
of the mother is modified by the above agents.

FORCEPS

The foundation for the remaining major obstetrical practices has
been set and it is therefore imperative to insure a live newborn.
Forceps are required with an incidence as high as 65% in some American
hospitals.[39] In "Williams Obstetrics" Chapter 40, entitled "Forceps,"
the authors state "all methods of analgesia interfere to a certain
extent with the mother's voluntary expulsive efforts, in which circumstances, low forceps delivery becomes the most reasonable procedure . .
. .low mid forceps . . has become extremely popular with the advent
and increasing use of conduction anesthesia."[40] When forceps have
been used to extract the fetus, those infants so delivered have an
increased incidence of intracranial hemorrhages, damage to the facial
nerve and brachial plexus with the potential of other neurological
impairment.[41] ·

EPISIOTOMY

Suzanne Arms gives a table of statistics of a large urban teaching hospital.[38] (Total deliveries 2,313; episiotomies 1,773 - 77%; forceps 629 - 27%; stimulated labor 1,032 - 45%; induced labor 284 - 12%; and Caesarian section 249 - 11%). The examples of almost all women receiving episiotomies has convinced them that no birth could occur without large, jagged tears of their perineal tissues, therefore necessitating the surgical intervention of an episiotomy. Episiotomy incorporates other obstetrical interventions including shaving of the perineum, local anesthetic, and an increase in post-partum hemorrhage. Nerves, muscles, and skin are severed causing numbness and discomfort months after delivery. In spite of the al-most universality in America concerning episiotomies, Holland's rate is only 8%. Deviation from the natural process continues as this surgical wound is repaired, requiring more anesthetic and thereby promoting neurological sequelae.

CONSEQUENCES OF NOT ENCOURAGING BREASTFEEDING

The World Health Organization, the American Academy of Pedia-trics, the American Public Health Association and other responsible medical authorities have all agreed that breastfeeding is the prime method of nourishing young babies. Despite this mandate, women in the United States receive little, if any, encouragement to nurse their infants.[43] Infant feeding practices in the United States have, thus, paralleled the unnatural course of obstetrical science. The entire labor and delivery process of preventive obstetrics has technologi-cally influenced infant feeding practices by substituting formulas for natural mother's milk - indeed, a "medical mastectomy." Although documentation medically, psychologically, sociologically, and econo-mically have yielded firm support for breastfeeding, most infants are bottle fed and consume commercial baby foods during the first or second month of life.[43]

Special attention has been drawn to the abandonment of breast-feeding in many developing nations. A recent report from the World Health Organization[44] noted the rise in the infant mortality rate in rural Chile; this rise coincided with the fall in the prevalence of breastfeeding. Documentation of the consequences of artificial feed-ing in the United States by Grulee et al. in 1935, Hausman et al. in 1974, and most recently summarized by Gerrard, 1974,[45] represents find-ings similar to those of the World Health Organization concerning the third-world nations.

Breastfeeding not only provides protein, calories, salts, vita-mins, and fluid, but fosters intimate physiologic and emotional rela-tionships between mother and child and involutes the uterus as well as providing protection against several gastrointestinal and respiratory pathogens.[43,45] The most convincing evidence was provided by the in-vestigations and surveys of Dr. Clifford G. Grulee, Professor of Pedia-trics, Rush Medical College, in the 1930s in Chicago. His was a study of 20,061 cases over nine months.

Grulee separated the 20,061 cases into three groups:[46]

GROUP 1 were entirely breastfed: 9,749 cases (48.5% of total) GROUP 2 were partially breastfed with accessory feedings: 8,605 cases   (43% of total) GROUP 3 were artificially fed: 1,707 cases (8.5% of total)

The morbidity of the groups was as follows with the artificially fed group clearly the highest, the partially fed group next, and the totally breastfed group the lowest:[46]

GROUP 3	63.6% morbidity
GROUP 2	53.8% morbidity
GROUP 1	37.4% morbidity

The mortality statistics are even more revealing. The average mortality of these infants per year was 1.1%. Of the total mortality there were nearly 10 times as many deaths among the artificially fed as among the totally breastfed. The percents of the total are as follows:[46]

GROUP 3	66.1% of the mortality
GROUP 2	27.2% of the mortality
GROUP 1	6.7% of the mortality

Colostrum, the fluid that lactating women produce during three to five days postpartum, is a rich source of antibodies, particularly secretory immunoglobulin A. Although the antibodies are poorly absorbed into the bloodstream, they work locally, offering protection against allergens and pathogens that enter the gastrointestinal tract.[43] None of the protective factors found in human milk is found in formulas. Recent studies have shown that cells within colostrum and human milk may protect premature infants from necrotizing enterocolitis.[47] The antimicrobial enzyme, lysozyme found in appreciable quantities in human milk offers a bacteriocidal effect on invading pathogens.[48] Dr. Paul György, one of the foremost clinical investigators on breastfeeding identified a group of nitrogen-containing polysaccharides, the bifidus factor, which promotes the growth of the bifido bacterial flora characteristic of breastfed infants. These acid-producing bacteria lower the pH of the gastrointestinal tract and subsequently may inhibit the growth of E. coli, yeast, & shigella organisms.[49] The protein lactoferrin also found in human milk has been implicated in preventing microbial infections by inhibiting the proliferation of staphylococci and E. coli (i.e., binds iron which the bacteria require for growth).[50] Lactoperoxidase, an anti-streptococcal factor, and another anti-staphylococcal factor (a fatty acid), are also included in the anti-infectious agents found in human milk.[51]

Other naturally acquired biochemical and physiologic benefits from human milk include the recommendation of human milk to the progeny of families with a history of allergy.[45] Since cow's milk allergy is the most common allergy of infancy, can one assume without presumption that cow's milk is for calves and human milk for infants?

Most recent research on the biochemical differences between human milk and cow's milk reveals a possible etiology of the increase of atherosclerosis and heart disease. Human milk contains ten times

more the amount of cholesterol than cow's milk formula. Evidence
from animal studies pertaining to this major biochemical difference
suggests that infants may require a moderate amount of dietary cholesterol to establish mechanisms for proper metabolism of cholesterol later in life.[52] Other research findings are in accord and im-
ply that low cholesterol formulas may contribute to atherosclerosis.[53]
The dangers and risks of deviation from the natural process of breastfeeding do not escape the artificially formula-fed infant. Overfeeding and too high a caloric intake have been implicated in precipitating excessive numbers of fat cells. Studies of overweight children
have revealed that a significantly high proportion had been overweight since early childhood. These children could be fated to a
lifetime of fighting obesity. The etiology of overfeeding infants
lies in the method - artificial with set feeding schedules. Not only
does the mother and/or nurse who feeds the infant control the volume
and concentration of the formula, but they also encourage drinking
the entire contents of each bottle. However, if the baby is naturally breastfed on demand and until satisfied, overfeeding and con-
sumption of unnecessary, detrimental calories does not result.[54,55]

DESPITE HUMAN MILK'S LOW COST, AVAILABILITY, PATHOGEN-FREE
STATE, AND MANDATORY IMPORT TO THE HEALTH OF NEWBORNS,
PEDIATRICIANS AND OBSTETRICIANS REMAIN SILENT ON ENCOURAGING
BREASTFEEDING THUS CONTRIBUTING DAILY TO THE MORBIDITY AND
MORTALITY OF THE WORLD, AND IF CONTINUED, WILL CONTRIBUTE TO
GENERATIONS OF PHYSICAL AND MENTAL PATHOLOGY NOT YET WITNESSED.

The Pan American Health Organization study[56] demonstrated that
breastfeeding protected babies against gastrointestinal tract and
nutritional diseases, but for the baby to be fully protected, human
milk had to be given alone, i.e., without additional cow's milk. The
economic waste of abandoning breastfeeding is considerable. It has
been projected that the feeding of a human milk substitute to one-
fifth of the children born in underdeveloped countries in urban areas
would cost $365 million per year. This sum does not include alloca-
tion of medical care funds to those infants who experienced the
dangers and risks of artificial feeding.[43] Despite human milk's low
cost, availability, pathogen-free state, and mandatory import to the
health of newborns, pediatricians and obstetricians remain silent on
encouraging breastfeeding. Their silence and inaction contribute
daily to the morbidity and mortality statistics of the world and, if
continued, will contribute to generations of physical and mental
pathology not yet witnessed.

ROUTINE HOSPITALIZATION

Routine hospitalization for birth, promoting "just-in-case"
and "exception-becoming-the-rule" obstetrical practices has not only
promoted pathology in both mother and infant, but has enforced rigid
separation of family members and long isolation of mother and infant
from siblings. Furthermore, these family-destructive forces not only
rob women of their natural function and raison d'être but also remove

humanism from the natural process. Homebirth is the natural choice
for those healthy women seeking an alternative incorporating healthy,
not pathological practices. Suzanne Arms states that the only reasonable argument against homebirth is that it is too simple and inexpensive a solution for such a complex society as ours.[38]

THE CHICAGO HOME OB SERVICE

The data to be presented here represent a study of childbirth
at home in a fee-for-service type practice in a carefully screened
varied urban metropolitan population of Chicago. The birth attendant
in this study was a physician (usually Mayer Eisenstein, MD) sometimes
accompanied by an assistant--a mother who has had homebirths of her
own and who has breastfed her babies. The attending physician is not
a specialist of *hospital-based* obstetrics, but rather of *home-based*
obstetrics. His training included the traditional four-year medical
school curriculum and one year of a rotating internship. Unique to
his education and training was a one-year apprenticeship to a home
delivery specialist and family medicine practitioner (Gregory White,
MD) whose experience includes approximately three thousand homebirths.
The writer participated as a preceptor in this study.

The essence of homebirth is affording a choice to a pregnant
woman. Her entry into the office signifies her decision - to deliver
her baby at home. At that moment an entire process, with the highest
priority given to health, is thereby initiated. It incorporates support systems: La Leche League International, pediatricians, family
practitioners, and most important, the family (including grandparents,
aunts, uncles, etc.).

SCREENING METHODS

The process and principles of selection, technique of prenatal
care, and management of labor, delivery, and puerperium will now be
discussed. Since the main requirement is that of a healthy woman,
the process is more precisely referred to as "criteria for exclusion."
These are obtained via personal discussion and include the following:

1. ## MEDICAL
    *   a previous medical history of symptomatic hypertension;
        renal, pulmonary and/or cardiac pathology; diabetes
        mellitus, or
    *   any previous or concurrent symptomatic systemic diseases.

2. ## SURGICAL
    *   a previous major hospital procedure pertaining to sur-
        gery of the uterus, cervix and/or vagina;
    *   subluxation of the femur, hip and/or vertebral column,
        requiring surgical reduction with resultant pelvic
        deformity;
    *   in some cases surgical consultation may be necessary
        in order to arrive at conclusive disposition.

3. OBSTETRICAL (which also includes several medical conditions with specific potential in affecting the outcome
   of parturition). Obstetrical criteria for exclusion
   would be a previous history including one or several of
   the following:

   * Caesarian section;
   * a baby weighing less than five pounds or greater than
     ten (a special judgement is given to this criterion,
     utilizing expert medical and obstetrical advice);
   * symptomatic toxemia including increased diastolic
     blood pressure greater than or equal to 90 mm Hg at
     term and persistent loss of sugar and/or protein in
     the urine;
   * hemorrhage during labor (i.e., abruptio placentae or
     placenta previa);
   * any long-term use of drugs, especially hormones with
     symptomatic findings, i.e., birth control pill with
     phlebitis and/or thromboembolism;
   * hemorrhage as a result of an intrauterine device;
   * conception despite the use of an IUD;
   * hemorrhage either previous, during, or after parturi-
     tion which required transfusion of blood;
   * dilation and curettage for abortion and/or miscarriage
     without normal delivery subsequently;
   * gross obesity, 20-25% greater than the ideal weight;
   * a hemoglobin of less than 10 grams and malnutrition;
   * any previous pregnancy with complications, either
     iatrogenically produced or of pathological etiology,
     is discussed and definitive judgement is reached under
     consultation on the safety of a homebirth.

4. MISCELLANEOUS
   * refusal to breastfeed;
   * no telephone;
   * a driving time of more than one and one-half hours from
     the Chicago Loop area, or to a hospital;
   * an anxious woman forced into choosing a homebirth because
     of fad, economics and/or outside pressures.

It is necessary to emphasize that the attending physician re-
serves the prerogative to arbitrarily exclude a woman as a potential
candidate for a homebirth.

PRENATAL CARE, EDUCATION, & PREPARATION

Almost all candidates for homebirth possess positive attitudes
and directions concerning health and nutrition. Therefore, extensive
dietary lists are not necessary; however, nutritional consultation is
available. Succinctly stated, we encourage all women to eat a nutri-
tive, balanced diet consisting of protein, fat, and carbohydrate.
Conventional prenatal care, involving active intervention by the physician, of well pregnant women is eliminated as the above concepts
are accepted and practiced.

During the woman's initial visit a general medical history is recorded. Complete physical examination with emphasis on the obstetric exam is performed. Laboratory tests are minimal and include an initial hemoglobin concentration, blood type, Rh, VDRL, and urinalysis. All prenatal visits involve discussion on questions concerning homebirth, pregnancy, breastfeeding, and health. Explicit "don'ts" are given and include smoking, drugs, and "junk" foods. As fetal development accelerates, the conventional obstetrical examination is performed, i.e., (1) palpation and auscultation of the uterus and its contents; (2) visualization and palpation of the cervix and vagina; (3) clinical evaluation of the bony pelvis; (4) palpation of the presenting part if the fetus is sufficiently large; and (5) examination of the vulva, perineum, anus, and rectum. Weight and blood pressure are also recorded and there is further discussion on symptoms of early pregnancy, exercise and general care. At all times during office visits, family, i.e., husband and children, are present during discussions and examinations.

A copy of La Leche League International's book, "The Womanly Art of Breastfeeding," is given to each family. Other books that may be given and/or strongly recommended include:

"Childbirth Without Fear" by Grantly Dick-Read, MD
"Commonsense Childbirth" by Lester Dessez Hazell
"Emergency Childbirth" by Gregory White, MD
"The Experience of Childbirth" by Sheila Kitzinger
"Husband-Coached Childbirth" by Robert Bradley, MD

Many of these would be available in libraries or local bookstores; all can be obtained through the I.C.E.A. Supplies Center, P.O. Box 70258, Seattle, Washington 98107. While serving to reinforce healthy practices and answer questions not discussed, such reading also promotes further questions.

Another important factor in the education of the mother is the contribution of the attending physician's assistant who, in this instance, has three children of her own--all delivered at home and nursed. She is an integral part of all discussions and an important resource for many questions.

The management of pre-natal care is preparatory for labor and homebirth. The obtaining of specific materials including rubber sheets, newspapers, large pots, towels, safety pins, flashlights, etc. are gathered by the expecting family. The necessary equipment, including drugs, i.e., synthetic oxytocin, meperidine, epinephrine, etc. almost all of which remains in two large satchels, is brought by the attending physician to the home. The estimated date of confinement is only an estimate and, therefore, the woman who is near or at term calls whenever pre-labor or labor has actually begun. An answering service with emergency long distance page and two other telephone numbers can be utilized to alert the physician. Support for overlapping deliveries is covered by two other homebirth specialist physicians in the Metropolitan Chicago Area.

THE HOME PHYSICIAN'S ROLE IN BIRTH

Preventive interferences and "just-in-case" routine laboratory examinations are eliminated during the prenatal care. The persistent theme of "natural childbirth through health" has been aspired to, and through delivery, becomes a reality. The natural process continues through labor, delivery, and the puerperium. A telephone call and/or page alerts the physician on the progress and events of labor. After arriving at the home, abdominal palpation, auscultation and a pelvic examination are performed. The presenting fetal part and its relationship to the bony pelvis, cervical os dilatation, effacement and status of the amniotic membranes are noted. Following the examination, the findings are explained to the expectant parents and, depending on the stage and progression of labor, the woman is free to continue her daily routine at home. It is important to note that we encourage eating and drinking, but not excessively. The laboring woman rests until strong uterine contractions interfere; either ambulation or standing is then advised. The couple, family and/or friends remain close and supportive throughout labor and delivery, as the attending physician becomes a consult to this natural process. Depending on the individual parturient and stage of labor, the delivery area is now complete with the attendants' obstetrical aids. Since time spent in a particular home may vary from two to twelve hours or more, the physician is permitted to experience this family in an intimate setting.

The second stage of labor with complete cervical dilation and effacement heralds strong uterine contractions with shorter intervals of rest. The physician remains in his consultant role, as supportive comforting measures, including ambulation and/or back and leg massage, etc. are performed by family members and/or friends. As the fetal head crowns and the perineal tissues are stretched, a variety of positions in preparation for actual birth are taken, and include semi-sitting, a left or right Sims (lateral) and/or squatting, depending on the mother's comfort. With the delivery of the newborn's head, instructions on controlling the subsequent contractions are given and delivery of the shoulders ensues conforming to the tortuous course of the birth canal.

THE ONLY REASONABLE ARGUMENT AGAINST HOMEBIRTH IS THAT IT IS TOO SIMPLE AND INEXPENSIVE A SOLUTION FOR SUCH A COMPLEX SOCIETY AS OURS.

SUZANNE ARMS

Emotions are at a peak as the new mother and father observe the first seconds of life, heralded by a cry. In the next 15 minutes the pulsations of the umbilical cord stop, the cord is cut, the infant is weighed, and the placenta is delivered as the third stage of labor is completed, with the father holding his child. The physician rapidly removes wet newspapers, sheets and towels; the new mother now stands and walks to a chair to begin nursing her infant. Perhaps the most crucial moment is the immediate post-partum period, and the natural process continues as the suckling infant stimulates further oxytocin secretion and thereby involutes the uterus and arrests post-partum hemorrhage.

Further instructions on nursing, newborn care and potential development of post-partum symptoms are given before leaving. The most important symptom is post-partum hemorrhage. In the event of the remote possibility that hemorrhage cannot be naturally controlled via breastfeeding, ergonovine maleate (Ergotrate) in the form of oral tablets is prescribed with proper instructions.

The family surrounds the nursing mother and newborn as we gather the equipment. Before leaving the physician encourages rest when the baby sleeps, and implores the new parents to call if there are any questions. He states that his assistant will come the next day to fill out birth certificates, examine the child, and answer questions pertaining to nursing, infant care, and managing a family with a newborn. We then depart carrying two large leather satchels.

Post-natal care is minimal as all the support systems have promoted a natural pregnancy, birth, and breastfeeding. The infant will nurse and receive all its necessary nutritional requirements from human milk; solids are introduced after six months as breast-feeding continues. The baby and mother may return for three or four post-natal visits. Physical examination of the infant and further questions and problems are discussed. The number of puerperal visits are minimal as mother and child do not require active care. The physician again becomes a consultant and advocate to the new family's health.

STATISTICS

The above process has yielded clinical obstetric data and several interesting and typical homebirth case studies. It is not the intent of this paper to compare hospital-based obstetrical practice with that of homebirth; however, some important conclusions with supportive data will be stated. During the five months of preceptorship the writer observed 56 homebirths. An extensive obstetrical log was kept and approximately 40 parameters were recorded for each home delivery. The following statistically summarizes these births.

The population studied from January 1, 1975, to June 1, 1975, formed a widely varied group socioeconomically and geographically in the metropolitan Chicago area.

1. 56 homebirths:

    50 White
    3 Mexican-American
    2 Black
    1 Oriental

2. Average age: 26.6 years

3. Number of pregnancies: Range: primagravida to 9 gravida

    primagravida   23.2%
    para 2   30.4%
    multipara   46.4%

4. Estimated date of confinement relative to the date of
    delivery: average = +3.3 days

5. Average weight gained: 30.2 pounds

6. Position of mother at time of delivery:

semisit	92.8%
Sims (lateral)	1.8%
hands & knees (i.e. breech)	3.6%
squat	1.8%

7. Position of fetus:

occiput anterior	94.6%
occiput posterior	1.8%
frank breech	3.6%

8. Amniotic membranes:

spontaneous rupture	82.1%
artificial rupture:	
1st stage	0.0
late 2nd stage	17.8%

9. Meconium staining:

light and questionable (4)	7.1%
definite (1)	1.7%

10. Artificial Uterine Stimulation:

Labor induction	0.0
Labor stimulation	0.0

11. Pre-delivery medication (1st & 2nd Stage):

analgesia	0.0
anesthesia	0.0

12. Delivery medication:

anesthesia	0.0

13. Episiotomy: 0.0

14. Tears requiring suture (2):   3.6%
         (both minimal and requiring two stiches each)

15. Extraction:

forceps	0.0
other maneuvers	0.0

16. Resuscitation of infant (1):   1.7%
         (use of DeLee suction device to evacuate mucus)

17. 3rd stage extraction of placenta: 0.0

18. Cervical tears: 0.0

19. Blood transfusions: 0.0

20. Death:

         maternal   0.0
         infant   0.0

21. Average birth weight: 8 pounds

22. Infant feeding:

         breastfeeding   100%
         artificial feeding   0.0

It should be noted that no delivering woman and/or infant required
hospitalization.

The above data exemplify   natural childbirth. Although the
numbers gathered are small, they indicate that healthy pregnant women can proceed through parturition without interference in the form
of obstetrical prophylaxis. If one promotes the natural process,
then the results yield health. Although the population studied
varies socioeconomically, a universal characteristic was observed--
all families had similar nutritional habits. Surreptitious inspec-
tion of cupboards, pantries and refrigerators in all homes yielded
evidence of supplies of fresh vegetables and fruits, lean mean and
fish, whole grain breads, cheeses, yogurt, and the comparative absence of store-bought processed foods. It can be concluded that pregnant women who eat a healthy balanced diet do gain weight and do
produce healthy babies with superior birth weights.

The value of natural homebirths is apparent through examination
of the process of noninterference. Let us examine the ramifications
of these processes and practices:

     * If the amniotic membranes remain intact without artificial
rupture, there is no excessive molding of the infant's head;
     * If intravenous routes are not set up, then mothers eat and
drink and do not develop acidosis;
     * If synthetic oxytocin for either stimulation and/or induc-
tion is not infused, then the need for analgesia and/or anesthesia
is all but eliminated and labor progresses naturally;
     * If analgesia and/or anesthesia is not administered, then
labor progresses naturally, normally, and without narcotization of
the newborn;
     * If the lithotomy position (i.e., stirrups) is not prescribed,
then labor progresses normally and need for drugs is all but eliminated and the delivery position is of free choice;
     * If episiotomies are not done, then post-partum hemorrhage,
nerve and muscle trauma are minimal;

If all of these practices are heeded, then forceps and other obstetrical maneuvers are unnecessary. Since all the statements previously delineated are documented and statistically supported, the end
result of healthy babies and families is not surprising.

CASE STUDIES

The following typical case studies are presented to illustrate and confirm the data and conclusions given above:

CASE STUDY NUMBER 1: M.P., 30 year old, white, para 1, gravida 2, EDC (estimated date of confinement) January 22, DD (date delivered) January 30, weight gain +39 pounds, delivery position SS (semisit), position of baby OA (occiput anterior), spontaneous rupture of membranes, NSVD (normal spontaneous vaginal delivery of baby & placenta), no drugs or obstetrical interventions. M.P. gave birth to a 7 lb, 8 oz girl, Apgar 10 at 1 min and 10 at 5 minutes. Previous medical history unremarkable, & physical examination was within normal limits; however, previous obstetrical history included a complicated premature delivery of her first child. She was told she had an abruptio placentae & that her baby was premature and infant was placed in an incubator for 2 days; mother and baby returned home seven days after admission.

M.P. described her first baby's delivery as a "terrible" experience. She states that the hospital was "too tense of an atmosphere ... too sterile ... felt like you're incapable of having a child ... they take you over ... no one listened to me ... the obstetrician did not get to the delivery ... ice chips not even permitted ... never held the baby ... placed in incubator ... could not nurse ... held baby for first time at two days of age ... baby missing."

REFLECTIONS & REMARKS: Baby's whereabouts unknown as nurse discovered that the infant was not with her mother. "Did I get my baby? ... what kind of mothering in an incubator? ... lack of mothering and tense hospital affected the baby ... could baby's colic be due to the hospital experience ... from the beginning of my pregnancy obstetrician was angry about weight gain of 3 pounds per month ... obstetrician had me on a low calorie diet ... became toxemic ... gained only 10-12 pounds during 1st pregnancy .. they told me I had abruptio placentae & that they saved my life ... went to a different obstetrician for 2nd baby; he reviewed my past and then said this delivery would be 'normal'; however, upon learning that I now planned a homebirth, he stated I was 'high risk' ... homebirth was biggest thrill of my life ... delivery was calm, comfortable and warm; my husband was close by ... since baby's life begins at birth, she needs all the love and care from the start, and we were there at all times and not separated ... my baby nursed immediately ... this baby's first months differed greatly from my older child's ... the older boy is tense and fearful ... this new baby appears so serene."

COMMENTS: This family lives on the south side of Chicago in a large restored late-19th century house. M.P.'s delivery was normal; however there was a mucosal tear of the perineum but did not require repair. We spent three hours at the house & enjoyed home-baked bread and herbal tea after delivery. Their food larder was filled with fresh vegetables and fruits.

CASE STUDY NUMBER 2: L.D., 24 year old, black, para 1, gravida 2, EDC February 1, DD February 7, weight gain +27 lbs, delivery position SS, position of baby OA, spontaneous rupture of membranes NSVD, no drugs or obstetrical interventions. L.D. gave birth to a 6 lb 2 oz girl, Apgar 9 at 1 minute and 10 at 5 minutes. Previous medical history unremarkable, previous obstetrical history includes a NSVD at home of a boy; physical examination within normal limits.

REFLECTIONS & REMARKS: Does not believe in hospitals "..institutions have too many trips to take you on ... very impersonal ... at home my family and friends are close."

COMMENTS: A large extended family living on the south side of Chicago. A strong African influence everywhere in the house, including art, music and food. We slept on African rugs after drinking herbal tea and eating home-made cookies. Her cupboards and shelves were filled with whole grained flour, dried beans, fruit & nuts. L.D. gave birth in her dress design studio on a large pattern table with family and friends surrounding and actively supporting her. Baby breastfed immediately for half-hour. Departed in the snow.

PHYSICIANS HAVE UNIQUE POWER AND THE ESTABLISHED CHECKS AND BALANCES ARE POOR, AT BEST,

CASE STUDY NUMBER 3: L.J., 29 year old, white, para 4, gravida 5, EDC February 17, DD February 10, weight gain +31 lbs, delivery position SS, position of baby OA, spontaneous rupture of membranes, NSVD, no drugs or obstetrical interventions. L.J. gave birth to a 9 lb 3 oz boy, Apgar 10 at 1 minute and 10 at 5 minutes. Previous medical history unremarkable, physical examination within normal limits. Previous obstetrical history includes 3 normal, uncomplicated hospital deliveries and one uncomplicated homebirth.

REFLECTIONS & REMARKS: "family is close ... I don't have to leave my children ... they participate in the birth of their new sister or brother ... they don't feel alone."

COMMENTS: L.J.'s husband, a switchman for the railroad, was on a run in Wisconsin. The home was in Harvey, IL, and it was snowing as we entered a quiet house in the afternoon. All of the children were napping as Mrs. J. prepared lunch for herself & then for us. We ate home-made bread of home-ground whole wheat, organic honey, and home-made peanut butter. The children slept as their mother awaited the arrival of her oldest daughter (age 6) from school. With the onset of 2nd stage, her children awoke and entered their parents' bedroom. They were all eyes, watching the birth of their new brother. The mother walked to the rocking chair in the front room and nursed her newborn. The other children touched and held their new brother. We prepared dinner for the children, and departed reluctantly.

These case studies represent a true sample of all the home-births of this study, each with their own individuality, happiness and health. These reports and data demonstrate unparalleled success in the management of childbirth. However, in order to achieve this success, certain qualifications are necessary. Among them, an extensive experience in homebirth is primary. This criterion dis-qualified all hospital-trained obstetricians and therefore board-certified obstetricians, in particular, whose total experience and education have been confined to a hospital. Their teachers have passed on "pearls" of uncritical obstetrical practices for genera-tions.

CONCLUSIONS

As obstetrics in the United States becomes more technological, the goal of full normal human development approaches obscurity. To-tal health with its somatic, sexual, neurological, and psychological aspects remains an unattainable and unavailable ideal. Obstetric prophylaxis, "just-in-case", and "exception-becoming-the-rule" are the realities. During present litigious times, and as public aware-ness increases concerning the dangers and risks involved in conven-tional hospital-based obstetrics, will these common delivery tech-niques impose legal hazards to physicians, leading to malpractice charges?[57]

Physicians have a unique power, and the established checks and balances are poor, at best. The risks and dangers present in all allopathic medicine are experienced only by the patient; malpractice awards and settlements do not compensate for the real damages. The physician is protected unlike other professionals; he escapes the jeopardy of a commercial jet pilot whose actions, or inactions, are an intimate part of his own life and death as well as those of his passengers. This model cannot apply to the physician, although such an image, alone, could immensely reduce the incidence of "iatrogeno-cide."[42]

The natural processes are the physicians' foundation, yet de-viation continues. Nature will take her course despite interference and will react with a pathologic product not fit for survival. The natural process and health demand a time to be born.

EDITORS' NOTE: Medical students, residents, interns, or physicians interested in home obstetrics should write to the American College of Home Obstetrics, Gregory White, MD, President, 664 N. Michigan Ave., Suite 600, Chicago, Illinois 60611. For a brief description of the ACHO see p.183 of this book.

CITED REFERENCES

1. Brody, Jane E., "Obstetrical Practices Draw Warning," New York
    Times April 10, 1975, p. 48. (Meeting in New York City of the
    American Foundation for Maternal and Child Health.)

2. Bradley, R.A., Husband-Coached Childbirth. New York: Harper &
    Row, 1965.

3. Mendelsohn, R.S., "Dangers and Risks of Medical Care, or, Is
    Medical Care Worth Delivering?" University of Illinois Urban
    Preceptorship Program, April 1, 1975.

4. Lubchenko, L.O. et al., "Intrauterine Growth as Estimated from
    Liveborn Birth Weight Data at 24-42 Weeks of Gestation," Obstet.
    Gynecol. 32: 793-800, 1963.

5. Hardy, J.B., Editorial: Birth Weight and Subsequent Physical
    and Intellectual Development, New Engl. J. Med. 289: 973-974, 1973.

6. Grunewald, P.,"Growth of the Human Fetus,I. Normal Growth and its
    Variation," Am. J. Obstet. Gynecol. 94: 1112-1119, 1966.

7. Weiss, W., and E.C. Jackson, Maternal Factors Affecting Birth
    Weight, Perinatal Factors Affecting Human Development (PASBS
    publication no. 185) Washington, DC, Pan American Health Organi-
    zation, 1969.

8. Brewer, T.H., "Unborn Babies," Today's Living, March, 1975.

9. Brewer, T.H., Metabolic Toxemia of Late Pregnancy: A Disease of
    Malnutrition. Springfield: Thomas, 1966.

10. Strauss, M.B., "Observations on the Etiology of Toxemias of Preg-
    nancy: Relationship of Nutritional Deficiency, Hypoproteinemia,
    and Elevated Venous Pressure to Water Retention in Pregnancy,"
    Am. J. of the Medical Sciences 190: 811, 1935.

11. Ross, R.A., "Relation of Vitamin Deficiency to the Toxemia of
    Pregnancy," Southern Medical J. 28: 120, 1935.

12. Strauss, op.cit.

13. Brewer, T.H., "Human Maternal-fetal Nutrition," Obstet. Gynecol.
    112: 440, 1972.

14. Butler, N.R. et al., Collaborative Perinatal Study at National
    Institute of Neurological Diseases and Stroke, 1969.

15. Brewer, T.H., "Consequences of Malnutrition in Human Pregnancy,"
    Perinatal Medicine, Ciba Review, 1975.

16. Kelsey, F.O., "Drugs in Pregnancy and Their Effects on Pre- and
    Post-Natal Development," Research Publications Associations for
    Research in Nervous and Mental Disease 51:233-243, 1973.

17. Newton, M., National Study of Maternity Care Survey of Obstetric Practice and Associated Services in Hospitals in the U.S.: A Report of the Committee on Maternal Health, The American College of Obstetricians and Gynecologists, Chicago, 1970.

18. Kelsey, F.O., op. cit.

19. ibid.

20. Sinclair, J.C., H.A. Fox and J.F. Lentz, "Intoxication of the Fetus by a Local Anesthetic," New Engl. J. Med. 273: 1173, 1965.

21. Guillozet, N., "The Risks of Paracervical Anesthesia: Intoxication and Neurological Injury of the Newborn," Pediatrics 55: 533, 1975.

22. Rosefsky, J.B., and M.E. Patersiel, "Perinatal Deaths Associated with Mepivacaine Paracervical Block Anesthesia in Labor," New Engl. J. Med., 278: 530, 1968.

23. O'Meara, O.P., and J.V. Brazie, "Neonatal Intoxication after Paracervical Block," New Engl. J. Med. 278:1127, 1968.

24. Greenwald, P. et al., "Vaginal Cancer after Treatment with Synthetic Estrogens," New Engl. J. Med. 285: 390, 1971.

25. Barber, H.R. et al., "Vaginal Adenosis, Dysplasia and Clear Cell Carcinoma after diethylstilbestrol Treatment in Pregnancy," Obstet. Gynecol. 43: 645-452, 1974.

26. Goodman, L.S., and A. Gilman, The Pharmacological Basis of Therapeutics, 4th Ed. New York: MacMillan Company, 1970.

27. Editorial: A Time to be Born, The Lancet, Nov. 16, 1974.

28. Caldeyro-Barcia, R. et al., "Fetal and Maternal Monitoring in Spontaneous Labors and in Elective Inductions: A Comparative Study," Am. J. Obstet. Gynecol. 120(3): 356-362, 1974.

29. Niswander, K.R., and R.J. Patterson, Obstet. Gynecol. 22:228, 1963.

30. ibid.

31. Caldeyro-Barcia, R., Perinatal Factors Affecting Human Development: Proceedings of the Special Session held during the Eighth Meeting of the Pan American Health Organization Advisory Committee on Medical Research, Scientific Publication No. 185, Washington, DC, 10 June, 1969.

32. ibid.

33. Scwarcz, R.L. et al., "Fetal Heart Rate Patterns in Labors with Intact and with Ruptured Membranes," J. Perinatal Med. 1:153, 1973.

34. Caldeyro-Barcia, R. et al., "Effects of Position Changes on the Intensity and Frequency of Uterine Contractions During Labor," Am. J. Obstet. Gynecol. 80:284, 1960.

35. "Supine Called the Worst Position for Labor, Delivery," Family Practice News," June 1, 1975, Vol 5, No. 11.

36. Adamson, K., H.O. Morishisma, and A.C. Commis-Urrutia, Factors Influencing the Acid-Base State of the Fetus during Labor, Proceedings of the Pan American Health Organization, as cited #31.

37. Bienarz et al., Radiographic Study of Lithotomy Position and Effects on Circulation, Proceedings of the Pan American Health Organization, as cited #31.

38. Arms, S., Immaculate Deception. San Francisco Book Company: Houghton-Mifflin, 1975.

39. Haire, D., The Cultural Warping of Childbirth. Milwaukee: International Childbirth Education Association, 1972.

40. Hellman, L.M. and J.A. Pritchard, Williams Obstetrics, 14th Ed. Meredith Corporation, 1971.

41. Hubinout, P. et al., "Effects of Vacuum Extractor and Obstetrical Forceps on the Fetus and Newborn: A Comparison. 5th World Congress of Gynecology and Obstetrics. Sydney, Australia, 1967.

42. Young, Q., Chairman, Department of Medicine, Cook County Hospital, neologism,"iatrogenocide" (iatrogenic genocide).

43. Hausman, P. et al., White Paper on Infant Feeding Practices. Center for Science in the Public Interest, Washington, DC, 1974.

44. Plank, S.J. and M.L. Milanesi, Bulletin of the World Health Organization 48:203, 1973.

45. Gerrard, J.W.,"Breastfeeding: Second Thoughts," Pediatrics 54(6), 1974.

46. Grulee, C.G., H.N. Sanford, and P.H. Heron, "Breast and Artificial Feeding. Influence on Morbidity and Mortality of Twenty Thousand Infants," JAMA 103:735, 1934.

47. Medical World News, September 27, 1974, p. 29.

48. Miller, T., J. Bacteriol. 98: 949, 1969.

49. György, P., Am. J. Clin. Nutrition 24: 970, 1971.

50. Hentges, D., J. Bacteriol. 93: 2029, 1967.

51. Bullen, J. et al., British Med. J. 1: 69, 1972.

52. Reiser, R., and Z. Sidemas, J. Nutrition 102: 1009, 1972.

53. Hahn, P., and L. Kirby, J. Nutrition 103: 690, 1973.

54. Fomon, S., Infant Nutrition, p. 79, 1974.

55. Hirsch, S., and J. Knittle, Federation Proceedings 29:1516, 1970.

56. Puffer, R.R., and C.V. Serrano, Patterns of Mortality in Child-
    hood, Scientific Publication No. 262, Pan American Health Orga-
    nization, W.H.O., 1973

57. Stimeling, G., "Will Common Delivery Techniques Soon Become
    Malpractice?", J. Legal Med., May, 1975.

HOMEBIRTHS AND THE PHYSICIAN
Mayer Eisenstein, MD, ACHO*

A real turning point in my life was the birth of our first child in a hospital. At that point, I really had no intention of moving in any direction of childbirth or breastfeeding. And my wife really didn't either. We were just interested in having a birth without drugs and to have our baby right away. But when I realized that this was becoming progressively impossible as the expected delivery day approached, we called Dr. Robert Mendelsohn. He came to the hospital when labor was in progress and when he arrived, the obstetrician left. The obstetrician didn't show up again until 5 minutes before our son was born. At that point we just wanted to leave the hospital as soon as possible and so we did--less than an hour after he was born. As we left, Dr. Mendelsohn said, "Why don't you call Dr. Gregory White and see what he is doing." I did and then proceeded to spend the next couple of months with him. After witnessing about one birth with Dr. White, I realized that the direction he had taken was the right direction. During the years since then, our last two children have been born at home and we have been really heavily involved with childbirth at home.

One of the reasons I was predestined to be involved with the childbirth movement is that my grandmother was 45 years old when my mother was born. And my mother was born at home with a midwife which, even at that time, was bucking the system that said "women over 30 should not have babies." My mother then turned around and I was born when she was only 16, also with a midwife in a home-like environment, in Shanghai, China. So I have in my family, in just two generations, such anti-establishment familial blood that it was impossible for me to really turn out any different.

I would like to begin with some comments on what I think is important in "prepared childbirth." I see a problem with some sorts of "prepared childbirth" because we don't always prepare people for the right things. Some of the mothers I have witnessed giving birth have had no formal "preparation" whatsoever and do better than some who have. So let me give you a couple of things I think are very important to be prepared for.

---

* MAYER EISENSTEIN is a Cofounder and Vice President of the American College of Home Obstetrics and is a private homebirth practitioner in the Chicago Area. The thoughts written here are taken from his verbal presentation at the First American NAPSAC Conference where, on a scant 24 hour notice, he graciously filled in for the scheduled speaker, Gregory White, MD. Dr. White could not come when the day before the conference it became evident that a mother whom he promised to attend, then two weeks beyond her EDC, might go into labor at any moment. He therefore had to meet this higher obligation and was not able to come speak. Dr. Eisenstein apprenticed under the tutorship of Dr. White and is currently Dr. White's partner. Hence, as Dr. White's student and associate, Dr. Eisenstein presents here much of the thought and philosophy Dr. White might have presented himself.

* GREGORY WHITE is a Cofounder and President of the American College of Home Obstetrics; author of the book, "Emergency Childbirth"; and Medical Advisor & Founding Father, La Leche League International.

Number one is nutrition. This is probably more important to the outcome of a pregnancy than the couple's preparation for the home delivery itself. Dr. Tom Brewer has emphasized this over and over again for years. If I had my choice of a thousand well-nourished women giving unattended homebirth versus a thousand malnourished women delivered by the utmost specialist in the country, I would place my money on those thousand unattended women to have healthier babies. Good nutrition is probably more important than a good physician. And until we get the importance of nutrition across this has to be our strongest message to prepared parents. This may sound like a harsh statement, but I would rather a woman be well-nourished during her pregnancy, knocked out during the delivery, and breastfeed the baby than a woman follow the advice of starvation diets and have so-called "natural childbirth" without drugs. Of course, I wouldn't want the drugs either, as such, but if those were the choices, that's the way I would choose. The effect on the baby of a few hours of drugs during delivery is not nearly as potentially damaging, in my opinion, as 9 months of poor diet in pregnancy. Until we really stress this there will be no real change in the medical advice given to, nor the eating habits of, expectant mothers.

> IF I HAD MY CHOICE OF A THOUSAND WELL-NOURISHED WOMEN GIVING UNATTENDED HOMEBIRTH VERSUS A THOUSAND MALNOURISHED WOMEN DELIVERED BY THE UTMOST SPECIALIST, FOR HEALTHIER BABIES I WOULD PLACE MY MONEY ON THE THOUSAND UNATTENDED WOMEN WITH GOOD NUTRITION.

You see, one of the problems is that nature intended children to be born alive, and irrespective of what you do they usually survive. And that is the reason why doctors in this country have been able to get away with the horrendous things that are done. It takes 30 years sometimes to find out some little change such as the recent discovery of the damaging potential of diethylstilbestrol.   But even though it's inexcusable, things like DES only affect a very minor amount of people while malnutrition affects millions.

If we just look at one statistic in the Scandinavian countries we see that the average birth weight there is close to eight pounds. In this country it is almost a pound less. So far as I have been able to discern, the one biggest difference between our two cultures is that the average birth weight gain in this country is only around 20 pounds while in the European countries it is between 30 and 50. We have a scale in our office for only one reason and that is when women come for their monthly checkups, we make sure that they *gain* weight and we discourage women who are not gaining weight. We have been keeping strict records on this. It's very interesting when we see what happens. The average weight gain in our practice has been around 35 pounds and the average birth weight has been exactly eight pounds.

I think this is essentially where prenatal care should be headed. Not toward rules about no sex during pregnancy, or the monthly blood pressure for finding rare exotic diseases (which we do anyway to give the image of being doctors) which really has very little effect on the fetal or maternal outcome when compared to the profound effects of diet.

Another thing is, we've eliminated the use of the word "natural childbirth." We don't believe it exists. There is just "childbirth." Instead of referring to the ideal as "natural childbirth" we just say there is "childbirth" and, then, there is the "warped childbirth" as Doris Haire has mentioned.

I also take exception to the implication that as doctors "all we look for is pathology." I do look for pathology. I look for it every time. That doesn't mean you're supposed to do anything if none exists. Dr. Delee coined a phrase about 50 years ago called 'watchful expectancy." As I see it the role of the birth attendant, whether a physician, a midwife, or whatever, is to be there to watch, not interfere, but to be the lifeguard at the pool. Thousands of people may be swimming every day and he doesn't do anything. He just sits on his seat watching and getting a nice suntan until something happens. His fee is well earned whether he ever jumps in the water or not because he was there just in case something does happen.

Dr. Delee also made another statement that I'd like to share with you. He was the founder of the Chicago Maternity Center in 1895 and he, more than any one physician in this country, has been responsible for the horrendous trends of the "extremes becoming the means." He was the one who introduced outlet forceps as routine for delivery. He was the one who introduced episiotomy. Just before he died he said that if he had his whole life to live over again, he would only do homebirths and nothing else. That's a kind of a profound statement to me, and one really from a true devoted doctor who realized that the majority of his work was probably going to do bad instead of good.

DR. DELEE, WHO INTRODUCED FORCEPS AND EPISIOTOMY AROUND THE TURN OF THE CENTURY, STATED, JUST BEFORE HE DIED, THAT IF HE HAD HIS WHOLE LIFE TO LIVE OVER HE WOULD DO HOMEBIRTHS AND NOTHING ELSE, REALIZING THAT THE MAJORITY OF HIS WORK WAS PROBABLY GOING TO DO BAD INSTEAD OF GOOD.

Next to good nutrition for the pregnant mother, there's another thing that is very very important and something we can't separate from home childbirth and that is breastfeeding. We will never accept a couple who will not breastfeed their baby. This is absolutely required.

Another very, very exciting and interesting thing we have found regards weight gain by the newborn. I was trained that it takes seven to ten days for a newborn to regain its birth weight and I believed it. For that reason, the first couple of years I was in practice I was afraid to buy a pediatric scale because I was convinced that breast-fed babies don't gain as well in the beginning. Well, after a while we started realizing that the babies were really gaining very well. And so we quickly bought the scale to be able to quantify this. We found that by one week they usually exceeded their birth weight by one-half to one full pound. We interpret this to be the result of no maternal separation. It is very interesting because of my own family where our son was born in the hospital and had separation for almost an hour and he had a real hard time gaining. But our next two children were born at home with no separation and gained marvelously. Now, our son was only separated for an hour which is really a short period of time. But that's how important I think the imprinting is and that's how excessively important it is. Any person who is planning to set up any type of hospital-like home center has to be very careful that the baby is not taken away from the mother.

Let me mention a few of the things we do in our homebirth practice in Chicago. The way Dr. White has always done deliveries is nice and slow, letting the baby deliver itself - Just being there to gently hold the baby as it comes out - No holding back and no pulling on the head. There is no reason not to let a baby take its own time in coming out even if it just sits in the birth canal for a few minutes. The baby's head can be born for 10 or 15 minutes before the rest of the body is born without any problems. It will rotate by itself - No need to pull the baby to rotate. Just gently making sure it will gently ease out, that's usually all you need do.

We never suction babies routinely. That is something that should not be done. That's wrong. You worry about it only if the baby is not breathing. The baby that's breathing spontaneously has no business being suctioned because the mucous secretions have a very positive effect. Newborns have a tendency once in a while to stop breathing and the mucus secretions actually are a stimulant to breathe. The babies start coughing and sneezing. Usually this disappears within the first couple of days as does the mucus. Also, if the baby is breastfed right away, colostrum has been shown to have enzymatic effect to break down the mucous secretions.

A word on tears of the perineum. A baby's head, being fairly large to come through the vagina, the woman does experience, as I've been told many times, a very sharp burning sensation, one that feels like everything is going to tear apart. But this is something that extremely rarely happens to a great enough extent to be concerned about. In fact, one of the studies show that the only way to get a third degree laceration (that's a tear into the rectum) is by doing an episiotomy or having some kind of operative intervention. Dr. White, with 30 years of experience, said he has never seen a third degree laceration in a natural delivery.

We always give the baby to the mother immediately after birth with the baby crying spontaneously. This is the type of scene I just love so much: Father and mother holding each other, kissing themselves seconds after the baby is born, them holding the baby. Now at this first contact, we do not necessarily encourage breastfeeding. When you look to the animal kingdom, all animals don't nurse their babies within the first minute or two. They first lick the babies and hold them. First they make the attachment, then they go ahead and nurse within a few minutes after birth. Another thing we have found valuable is to make sure that every woman gets up right after the baby is born, preferably within the first few minutes. I don't like to see women nursing in bed right away because she needs to move. Lying down or sitting for a long time causes stasis of the blood while moving prevents blood clots afterwards.

I have shared with you some of the practices and attitudes we hold in our area with our homebirths. In closing I would like to make a statement regarding professional support for physicians who are sympathetic toward home childbirth and for physicians who would like information, education or training in the specialty of home obstetrics.

THE AMERICAN COLLEGE OF HOME OBSTETRICS

About six months ago a group of physicians, including myself, felt that there was a need for an organization. Initially, this organization was supposed to be a little club, one that met at the different people's houses every month where one of us would have prepared some literature research into some aspect of obstetrics, particularly as it concerns home obstetrics. In Chicago, we are very fortunate. I have three of the finest teachers in the country and it is because of them that I am here today. One is Dr. Robert Mendelsohn, another being Dr. Gregory White, and the other Dr. Herbert Ratner. It is because of their guidance that in Chicago we are able to do this. So we formed an organization called the American College of Home Obstetrics. I would now like to present to you our goal and our purpose and if there are any interested physicians, interns, or medical students, please let us know and we will send you some literature:

THE AMERICAN COLLEGE OF HOME OBSTETRICS has been founded to gather together those physicians who wish to cooperate with families who choose to give birth in the home, the natural and traditional place for birth throughout the world and the ages.

We also wish to learn from and teach each other the art of the safe supervision of home births. Members and Fellows are guided by an awareness that pregnancy, labor, and delivery are normal, physiological processes, not pathological events.

We rely on natural processes whenever feasible, reserving operative intervention of any kind or magnitude and, the giving of medication, for those cases where there is probability of damage to mother or baby without such intervention.

We take our ethic from the Hippocratic Oath & the World Medical Society Declaration at Geneva.

We try to foster, not only the welfare of our patients, mother and baby, but that of the entire family.

AMERICAN COLLEGE OF HOME OBSTETRICS
2821 Rose Street
Franklin Park, IL 60103
(312) 455-4286

Statistical Outcomes of Homebirths in the U.S.: Current Status

Lewis E. Mehl, MD*

We began our studies on the statistical outcomes of home deliveries because of the tremendous rise in the number of home deliveries
occurring across the country and the lack of any available data on
their outcomes. We had hoped to provide data which parents and professionals could use on their individual scales of relative value
along with the experiential data on emotional outcomes as they weighed
the risks and benefits to determine what kind of delivery they would
choose.

First, I will report the statistical outcomes of 1146 planned
homebirths in the San Francisco Bay Area and then I will compare this
to 180 similarly selected hospital deliveries performed by one of the
same groups of physicians. This is part of some ongoing work in which
we are attempting to accumulate a matched hospital series with which
to compare the home delivery statistics.

Our sources of data (Mehl, et al.,1976)[11] were the medical
charts from five home delivery services in northern California. The
five services included 3 physician groups and 2 lay midwife groups
as follows:

(1) A rural-based family practice in Western Marin County (Point
Reyes) composed of 3 family physicians and 3 registered
nurses, performing both home and hospital deliveries since
1970 as part of a comprehensive family practice.
(2) An urban-based family practice in Mill Valley composed of
2 physicians and 2 registered nurses--one a maternity nurse
practitioner--in practice since 1973.
(3) An urban-based group in Berkeley consisting of 1 physician
(whose training had been in pediatrics/neonatology) and 2
registered nurses, affiliated with a women's health cooperative in Berkeley. This group did not have hospital privileges and performed only home deliveries, referring women
requiring hospital care to local obstetricians. They had
been functioning since early 1974.
(4) 10 lay midwives from Santa Cruz County, functioning in both
urban and rural settings without immediate medical supervision, and with limited medical backup, performing births
since 1971.
(5) A rural lay midwife (Nancy Mills) from Sonoma County with
good physician backup, performing births since 1970.

* *LEWIS E. MEHL is Director of Research for the Institute for
Childbirth & Family Research and is author or coauthor of more
than 25 articles, book chapters and other works in the field of
Maternity care, family life, and psychiatry.*

In the latter service, records had been kept only for the last 171 of
her estimated 500 deliveries during a five year time span. All records
until April, 1975, were reviewed by one of us (LEM). They were adequately detailed regarding prenatal care, intrapartum and post partum
events, and infant and maternal follow-up. The groups represented the
following percentages of the total sample:

    (1) The Point Reyes physician group: 40.4%
    (2) The Mill Valley physician group: 11.2%
    (3) The Berkeley physician group: 7.6%
    (4) The Santa Cruz County midwives group: 30.8%
    (5) The Sonoma County midwife: 10.0%

The lay midwife from Sonoma County (Nancy Mills) began her midwifery activities accidentally, visitng a friend in labor. Others
learned she had attended a birth and asked her to their deliveries,
until she eventually developed a reputation as a midwife (See the
Chapter by Nancy Mills later in this book for more details on her
midwifery experience). Her training was self-acquired through reading and experience. The Santa Cruz midwives began functioning in much
the same fashion, becoming midwives to meet an experienced need in the
community, and educating themselves through discussion groups, experience, and reading. Their average fee per birth was $35.00, so that
their motivation was clearly not monetary. Typically, they were women
who had had an unattended homebirth and had decided to help other women avoid their predicament. The Sonoma County midwife had good medical backup through physicians (mainly family practice residents) at
the Community Hospital of Santa Rosa, who, while unwilling to attend
home deliveries, were willing to discuss problems over the telephone
and handle complicated deliveries in the hospital. The Santa Cruz
group had poor medical backup, and were not able to obtain telephone
consultation. They were often heavily criticized and condemned when
bringing women to the hospital who needed hospital care, and had few
supportive physicians to whom they could refer women with complications.
Labors in the Sonoma area were occasionally as far as one hour from a
hospital, although the usual distance was approximately 15 minutes.
Labors in the Santa Cruz area were occasionally as far as 45 minutes
from a hospital, but usually ranged from 5 to 15 minutes. Transport
facilities for both lay midwife groups consisted of the midwife's car
without any specialized support equipment. Equipment present at deliveries with the lay midwives was also minimal and typically consisted
of a bulb syringe, sterile gauze, sterile gloves, a fetoscope, blood
pressure cuff, urine dipsticks for testing acetones, glucose, and protein, a portable scale, and little else. Their mode of operation has
been described by Lang.[10]

The physician services brought a home delivery kit with them to
births. Typically the nurse would attend the labor from its inception
and the physician would arrive during the second stage for primigravidae and late first stage for multigravidae. The physician kit included IV equipment, oxytocin and Methergine for use after delivery,
other emergency drugs, forceps to use if necessary, as well as suture
supplies. (However, there was no intravenous oxytocin or forceps
used at home in this series.) The only equipment or drugs not present
in their kit and usually present in the hospital was whole blood. A

complete list of supplies is available on request (see addresses of authors tabulated at end of book). The transport vehicle for the physician groups was also the car belonging to the birth attendant. For the Point Reyes group, the closest hospital was 20 miles. For the Berkeley and Mill Valley groups the distance from a hospital was usually 5-10 minutes.

Prenatal care was essentially the same for all groups and did not deviate from the standards recommended by the American College of Obstetrics and Gynecology with regard to visit frequency, laboratory tests, and clinical assessment. The lay midwife groups required a minimum of two visits to a physician at which time clinical pelvimetry, Rh status, blood type, rubella titre, hemoglobin, hematocrit, VDRL and gonorrhea culture were determined. Nutrition, the avoidance of prenatal medication, and the psycho-social aspects of pregnancy were stressed more than is typically done in prenatal care, and visits usually lasted 20-30 minutes for the physician groups involving discussions with the nurse and then the doctor. For the lay midwife group, the visits were typically 30-60 minutes. Three women had no prenatal care, and first presented themselves in labor.

There was no limiting of weight gain. It was felt that every woman should gain at least 20-30 lbs. during pregnancy and the average weight gain was in the 30-35 lb range. Women with chronic medical disease were encouraged to seek a hospital, as were women who remained anemic. The threat of a hospital birth usually increased patient compliance with iron-containing preparations and, as a result, the number of women delivering at home with hemoglobins of less than 11.0 gm% was minimal (less than 1%).

Intrapartum care was essentially similar among the groups as well. The lay midwife groups did not perform breech or twin deliveries at home. The physician groups did, on occasion, although only after explaining the problems inherent in such deliveries. After 1973 the usual policy was to recommend Cesarean section to women with low breech scores (Zatuchni-Andros breech score) and to attend women with breech scores indicating safe vaginal delivery at home if the women so desired and requested. (Since the completion of this study, the lay midwives have begun attending some breech deliveries at home because of parents' dissatisfaction with the rising incidence of Cesarean section in the breech presentation.)

Labor prolongation, of itself, was not treated as a complication requiring hospitalization. Uterine inertia was initially often treated with buccal oxytocin by the physician group at home, and if results were not forthcoming, the woman was transported to the hospital for IV oxytocin. Prolongation of the second stage of labor was also not treated as a complication; indeed, most of the practitioners felt that a slower second stage with little pushing by the mother (often 2-3 hours) was *preferable* to a shorter second stage (less than 2 hours) characterized by an intense pushing effort by the mother. Cases of second stage arrest, however, if not responsive to buccal oxytocin over a 1-2 hour period, were transported to the hospital for forceps delivery. The midwives were unable to administer oxytocin and, consequently, sent more of their patients to the hospital for dystocia.

LAY MIDWIVES HAVE BEGUN ATTENDING SOME BREECH DELIVERIES AT
HOME BECAUSE OF PARENTS'DISSATISFACTION WITH THE RISING
INCIDENCE OF CESAREAN SECTION IN THE BREECH PRESENTATION.

Both groups monitored the fetal heart rate closely throughout
the first and second stage, using a fetal stethoscope or Doppler ultrasound fetoscope, and felt that any significant drop in heart rate
requiring intervention would be noticed. Blood pressures were checked
approximately every 1-2 hours during labor. Fetal heart tones were
checked as often as after every contraction during second stage if
some variability had been noted or if the mother were pushing particularly hard, but usually were taken every 15 minutes during second
stage and every 25-40 minutes during first stage, depending on the
character of the labor and the fetal heart rate pattern. The fetal
heart was occasionally listened to through a contraction and for some
time afterwards to determine the presence of any abnormal pattern.

Meconium staining without fetal heart rate irregularities was
not treated. (Meconium staining *with* fetal heart rate irregularities
was cause for hospitalization, and the infants, with one exception,
were treated with intubation and lavage.) Prolonged rupture of membranes in a term sized infant was followed, but not treated unless
necessary. It was felt that if the mother did not show signs of
amnionitis and had a good socioeconomic/nutrition background, that
intervention was not necessary within 24 hours. If labor had not begun by 24 hours, induction in the hospital was usually undertaken.

The midwives practiced perineal massage to prevent tearing,
while the physicians typically did not. This was optimally done by
the mother and father for the month prior to delivery and was done by
the midwife during the last half of the second stage. This was not
done consistently by all parents or all midwives, but it was felt by
the midwives that it helped prevent lacerations during delivery.

Forceps deliveries were not conducted at home, and no analgesia
or anesthesia was administered at home. If the latter was desired,
hospital transport was necessary for the woman to receive it.

The room in which the delivery occurred was kept warm and the
baby was given to the mother immediately after delivery to hold and
nurse, with blankets being placed around the infant to prevent heat
loss. The umbilical cord was not clamped until it ceased pulsating
except in Rh negative mothers, in whom it was clamped immediately
after delivery. RhoGam was given to the Rh negative mothers within 48
hours. Silver nitrate was *not* applied routinely to the infants' eyes
unless there had been a past history of gonorrhea, or one or both parents were unsure of the other. Most of the infants were fed only by
breast without glucose or formula supplementation, and were fed ad lib.

Home visits were usually made each day for the first three postpartum days, and telephone contact was maintained with the couple. The
infants were seen by the physicians at one week in their offices and
again at four weeks. After that point, the recommendations for well

child care of the American Academy of Pediatrics were observed. Midwives referred infants for newborn care after the first week to pediatricians or family physicians, and continued to follow the infants
themselves for varying periods of time. All mothers had a postpartum
examination from 4-6 weeks by a physician, and for the lay midwives,
results of this examination were recorded in their records.

STUDY POPULATION

Hazell[8] has described the demographic characteristics of the
homebirth population in the San Francisco Bay Area in a study of 300
home deliveries from the socioanthropological standpoint. Her subjects
overlapped to some extent with our sample and were derived from the
same subject pool--San Francisco Bay Area couples planning homebirth.

TABLE 1
HOME DELIVERY STUDY POPULATION

Contacted Home Delivery Service:	1,348	100.0%
Screened Out, Medical Dx	55	4.1%
Decided Against	147	10.9%
Attempted Home Delivery:	1,146	85.0%
Physicians	685	59.8%
Midwives	461	40.2%
Taken to Hospital:	136	11.9%
Physicians	58*	5.1%
Midwives	78*	6.8%
Completed Home Delivery	1,010	74.9%

* Patients hospitalized represented 8.5% of physicians'
cases, 16.9% of midwives' cases.

In Hazell's study, 90% lived in typical American fashion, with the
father gainfully employed, in a single family dwelling with one or two
cars, were not members of an ethnic minority, not on welfare, and
without household servants. A general characteristic of the group was
described as a self awareness shown in a concern for nutrition, health
foods, ecology, humanistic psychology, and a strong feeling for a natural birth process. Typically, the mother and father had both attended
college, but neither had graduated. The fathers' occupations were
noted to vary through the range of occupations present in the Bay Area,
from auto mechanic to physician to homesteader. Only one tenth were
classified as "hip," in rebellion to "normal American values," living
in a variety of alternative styles.

In our study, patients of the lay midwives tended to belong more
to the counter-culture than Hazell's population. In the physician
groups, more professional couples were included. A detailed socioeconomic study on one of the lay midwife groups (the Sonoma County
sample) is currently being coordinated by one of us (WEH), and a
psychological/developmental outcome study on a subsample of the Santa
Cruz group is being analyzed by two of us (LEM and GHP).

Table 1 (p. 77) presents statistics on the selection of the study population. Only 4% of those women who requested a home delivery were screened out for medical reasons (including premature labor, toxemia, and underlying systemic disease). This low percentage would seem to indicate that women seeking home deliveries are a self-selected healthy group, probably knowledgeable about childbirth, and the importance of nutrition in pregnancy. Nine women with previous fetal deaths were included in the homebirth sample. Previous obstetrical complications (with the exception of Ceasarean section) were not used as screening criteria, since it was felt that these were, to some extent, iatrogenic.

11% of the women who considered home delivery decided against it for non-medical reasons. This was highest in the lay midwife groups and may have been related to a hesitation to deliver without physician backup. In the physician-directed services, a common reason cited for switching to a hospital birth was that Medicaid would cover only hospital deliveries.

TABLE 2
CHARACTERISTICS OF MOTHERS

	Number	Percent	Calif 1973
Mother's Age:	1,146	100.0%	100.0%
< 20	60	5.2	17.3
20-34	1,068	93.2	77.6
≥ 35	18	1.6	5.1
Parity:	1,146	100.0%	100.0%
para 0	729	63.6	43.3
para 1	237	20.7	31.0
para 2	128	11.2	13.3
para 3	34	3.0	6.0
para ≥ 4	18	1.6	6.3
Prenatal Care Began:	1,146	100.0%	100.0%
1st trimester	707	61.7	72.8
2nd trimester	362	31.6	20.2
3rd trimester	74	6.5	4.5
none	3	0.3	2.4*

*includes prenatal care unknown

Of the 1,146 women beginning labor at home with the intention of delivering there, 136 (11.9%) were sent to the hospital to complete their delivery for treatment of intrapartum (11%) or postpartum (0.9%) problems. 88% of the deliveries begun at home were completed there. Thus, of the initial set of women contacting the home delivery services, 75% successfully delivered at home.

Four surviving infants required hospitalization for other than phototherapy within 3 days of delivery; a fifth was born very prematurely in the hospital, and remained there for one month.

Table 2 (p. 78) presents characteristics of the mothers and compares them to California statistics for 1973.[14] Over 90% were in the optimal childbearing age of 20-34 years, the average being 24.9 years. There was a high number (64%) of primigravidae in this series, and an incidence of grand multiparity of less than 1%. Virtually all of the women were trained in childbirth classes such as Bradley or Lamaze. 1145 women attempted breastfeeding (i.e., all but 1 of the series of 1146 total) and at 6 months of age 1138 were successful (i.e., 99.4%). These women tended to begin prenatal care later than the California 1973 sample, perhaps because they felt more knowledgeable and therefore, less of a need.

TABLE 3
CHARACTERISTICS OF PRESENTATION & DELIVERY

Presentation:	1,146	100.0%
Vertex	1,125	98.2%
Brow	(3)	(0.3%)
Shoulder	(3)	(0.3%)
Breech	21	1.8%
Delivery:	1,146	100.0%
Cesarean	28	2.4%
Vaginal	1.118	97.6%
Analgesia only	(14)	(1.2%)
Anesthesia only	(3)	(0.3%)
Both	(6)	(0.5%)
None	(1,095)	(95.5%)
Oxytocin:		
1st & 2nd Stage Labor	85	7.4%
3rd Stage Labor	235	20.5%
Forceps:		
Low Forceps	11	1.0%
Mid Forceps	6	0.5%
Perineal lesions:		
Lacerations Requiring Repair	148	12.9%
Episiotomies	89	7.8%

Table 3 (above) presents statistics on the presentations and deliveries. Most of the deliveries were vertex presentations (98.2%). Of the 21 breech presentations (1.8%) 10 delivered successfully, by choice, at home, while 11 were taken to the hospital. The latter were all unexpected and with lay midwives.

1% of the women studied had low forceps deliveries, 0.5% had mid forceps deliveries, and 2.4% were delivered by primary Cesarean section. The California Cesarean section rate was 9.9% in 1973. If, as the Mayo Clinic[1] found, half of the Cesarean sections are repeats, then California's primary section rate would approximate 50% (or double) the rate of this study.

OF THE 1,146 HOMEBIRTHS OF THIS STUDY, ONLY 8% HAD EPISIOTO-
MIES AND ONLY ANOTHER 13% HAD TEARS IN NEED OF REPAIR; THE
LOWEST INCIDENCE OF TEARING WAS AMONG LAY MIDWIVES, ONLY 5%, WHILE
IT WAS 40% AMONG THE HOMEBIRTHS ATTENDED BY PHYSICIANS.

Lacerations requiring repair were lowest (4.4% and 5.7%) in
the lay midwife groups and highest (40.2%) in the physician group
with the shortest experience in performing home deliveries without
episiotomies. Similarly, episiotomies were much lower for the lay
midwife groups than for the physician groups.

TABLE 4
INDICATIONS FOR THE 45 C-SECTIONS & FORCEPS DELIVERIES
IN THE 1,146 WOMEN BEGINNING LABOR AT HOME

LOW FORCEPS DELIVERY

Protracted descent	6
Arrest of descent	2
Dysfunctional labor	1
Brow presentation with arrest of descent	1
Fetal heart drop	1
	11

MID FORCEPS DELIVERY

Protracted descent	3
Arrest of descent	1
Dysfunctional labor	1
Fetal heart drop, occiput posterior (OP) presentation	1
	6

C-SECTIONS

Cephalopelvic disproportion (CPD)	16
Failure to descend, OP presentation, relative CPD	6
Arrest of active dilation, fetal heart drop, cord 4x neck	1
Prolapsed cord	1
Breech with amnionitis	1
Psychotic reaction to labor	1
Acutely dropping fetal heart tones	1
Toxemia	1
	28

Analgesia and/or anesthesia were used in only 2% of the vaginal
deliveries. During the first and second stage of labor, 38 women (or
3.3%) received buccal oxytocin at home, while 47 women (or 4.1%) received IV oxytocin in the hospital. Following completion of the third
stage of labor, 146 mothers received oxytocics at home (given entirely
by the physician group), 89 in the hospital. The mean length of first
stage was 10.2 hours for primigravidae and 4.6 hours for multigravidae;
second stage means were 118 and 45 minutes respectively. Table 4
(above) presents the indications for forceps deliveries and Cesarean
sections in the women beginning labor at home. There were 23 C-sections for cephalopelvic disproportion, 1 for fetal distress, 1 for toxemia, 1 for amnionitis, and 1 for psychotic reaction to labor.

TABLE 5
COMPLICATIONS OF LABOR & DELIVERY
(INDIVIDUAL WOMEN MAY BE LISTED UNDER MORE THAN 1 COMPLICATION)

| PRIMIGRAVIDAE (N=136/729=18.6%) | | | | |
Complication	Home	Hosp	Total	Percent[1]
Intrapartum				
Dystocia[2] 1st stage	27	34	61	8.4%
Dystocia 2nd stage	10	14	24	3.3
CPD	0	23	23	3.2
Meconium stain, only	24	3	27	3.7
FHT↓(c̄,s̄ meconium)	6	13	19	2.6
Hypertension	3	6	9	1.2
Brow presentation	1	2	3	0.4
Shoulder dystocia	1	1	2	0.3
Polyhydramnios	0	2	2	0.3
Other*	1	10	11	1.5
TOTALS	73	108	181	
Postpartum				
Hemorrhage[3]	1	3	4	0.5%
Excessive PP Bleeding[3]	11	7	18	2.5
Retained Placenta	10	4	14	1.9
Endometritis	9	2	11	1.5
PP Depression	0	4	4	0.5
TOTALS	31	20	51	

| MULTIGRAVIDAE (N=78/417=18.7%) | | | | |
Complication	Home	Hosp	Total	Percent[1]
Intrapartum				
Dystocia[2] 1st stage	2	12	14	3.4%
Dystocia 2nd stage	4	9	13	3.1
Meconium stain, only	11	1	12	2.9
FHT↓(c̄,s̄ meconium)	3	4	7	1.7
Precipitous labor	7	0	7	1.7
Other†	1	2	3	0.7
TOTALS	28	28	56	
Postpartum				
Hemorrhage[3]	4	1	5	1.2%
Excessive PP Bleeding[3]	9	4	13	3.1
Retained placenta	4	4	8	1.9
Endometritis	3	1	4	1.0
PP Depression	0	1	1	0.2
TOTALS	20	11	31	

* single cases of oligohydramnios, amnionitis, toxemia, prolapsed cord, thrombophlebitis, placenta previa, placenta abruptio, dehydration, urinary tract infection, 2nd trimester bleeding, and precipitous labor.

† single cases of cephalopelvic disproportion (CPD), shoulder dystocia, oligohydramnios.

1 Percent complications per 729 primigravidae, 417 multigravidae.
2 Dystocia is defined here as: prolonged or arrested 1st stage, failure to dilate, prolonged or arrested 2nd stage, failure to descend. (as per Greenhill & Friedman)
3 Hemorrhage is defined as more than 650 ml; excessive as "more than normal" including 3rd day postpartum bleed

Table 5 (p. 81) presents complications of labor and delivery in the homebirths of this study. (Individual women may be listed under more than one complication.) Interestingly, the total number of recordable events are comparable for primigravidae and multigravidae. The majority of the intrapartum problems involved first stage dystocia. However, the total incidence of protracted labor in this series is noticeably low when compared to the literature[6] as are meconium staining and fetal heart irregularities.[6,7] The overall incidence of 1st stage labor difficulties was 6.5%. The incidence of second stage problems was 3.2%. Often, the woman with second stage difficulties had also had first stage difficulties so that these numbers are not additive. Meconium staining occurred at a rate of 3.4% compared to 10-15% reported by Klaus & Fanaroff[9] for hospital populations. The incidence of fetal heart rate problems was 2.3%. Postpartum hemorrhage occurred at a rate of 0.8%, over half of which were managed successfully at home. Of the 4 postpartum hemorrhages transported to the hospital, all were by the lay midwife groups who could not carry oxytocin and IV supplies. Postpartum infection occurred at a rate of 1.3% and postpartum depression at a rate of 0.4%--all of which had been transported to the hospital for other reasons. There was no maternal hypotension prior to or during delivery.

Table 6, on the opposite page, compares the complications of labor and delivery between physicians and midwives. The lay midwives took more women to the hospital for induction of labor for prolonged rupture of membranes, uterine inertia during the first stage of labor fear to complete the delivery at home, falling fetal heart rate, manual removal of placenta and for treatment of postpartum hemorrhage. The physician groups used significantly more oxytocin after delivery of the placenta than the midwives, and reported more precipitous deliveries. There were no other differences between the two groups.

POSTPARTUM HEMORRHAGE OCCURRED ONLY 9 TIMES IN 1,146 BIRTHS AT HOME (0.8 %) AND WERE SUCCESSFULLY MANAGED IN ALL CASES; 5 OF THEM WERE MANAGED AT HOME AND 4 IN THE HOSPITAL.

These figures represent the course of events in those labors that were transported to the hospital. Table 7 (pp. 84-85) compares the complications observed between physicians and midwives. That the only differences were in the number of precipitous deliveries reported and in the amount of oxytocin used after the delivery of the placenta suggests that the powers of observation of the midwives equaled that of the physicians.

TABLE 6
COMPLICATIONS OF LABOR & DELIVERY
A COMPARISON BETWEEN PHYSICIANS & MIDWIVES
(INDIVIDUAL WOMEN MAY BE LISTED UNDER MORE THAN 1 COMPLICATION)

Complication	Physicians (N=134/685=19.6%)		Midwives (N=80/461=17.4%)	
	Number	Percent[1]	Number	Percent[1]
Intrapartum				
Dystocia[2] 1st stage	47	6.9%	28	6.1%
Dystocia 2nd stage	24	3.5	13	2.8
CPD	14	2.0	10	2.2
Meconium stain only	28	4.1	11	2.4
FHT↓($\bar{c},\bar{s}$ meconium)	16	2.3	10	2.2
Hypertension	7	1.0	2	0.4
Brow presentation	2	0.3	1	0.2
Shoulder dystocia	1	0.1	2	0.4
Polyhydramnios	1	0.1	1	0.2
Oligohydramnios	1	0.1	1	0.2
Precipitous labor	8	1.2	0	0.0
Other	6*	0.9*	3†	0.6†
TOTALS	155		82	
Postpartum				
Hemorrhage[3]	5	0.7%	4	0.9%
Excessive bleeding[3]	19	2.8	12	2.6
Retained placenta	15	2.2	7	1.5
Endometritis	10	1.5	5	1.1
Depression	3	0.4	2	0.4
TOTALS	52		30	

* single cases of amnionitis, placenta previa, abruptio placentae, dehydration, urinary tract infection, 2nd trimester bleeding.

† single cases of toxemia, prolapsed cord, thrombophlebitis.

[1] percent complication for 685 physicians' patients, 461 midwives' patients.

[2] see TABLE 5.

[3] see TABLE 5.

TABLE 7
REASONS FOR TRANSPORTATION TO THE HOSPITAL & THERAPY APPLIED

COMPLICATION & THERAPY	M.D.'s N=58*	Midwives N=78*	Stat. Sign.†
1st Stage Complications			
No prenatal care			
Dehydration→IV Hydration	1	0	NS
Severe Toxemia→Cesarean	0	1	NS
Prolonged rupture of membranes→Induction	0	4	p 0.01
Dystocia 1st stage (excluding CPD)			
Uterine inertia Oxytocin	7	19	p 0.001
Labor prolongation with↓FHT→			
Internal monitor & Oxytocin	1	0	NS
Arrest of Dilation			
Involving↓FHT & uterine inertia→			
Internal monitor & oxytocin	1	0	NS
Brow presentation→Oxytocin &			
low forceps	1	0	NS
Arrest & Uterine inertia→Oxytocin			
& low forceps	0	2	NS
Arrest→CPD, Cesarean	10	7	NS
Arrest→FHT, nuchal cord x4, C-sec	1	0	NS
Hypertension→			
Rx'ed with magnesium sulfate	1	0	NS
Untreated	5	0	NS
Bleeding during labor→No treatment	1	0	NS
Amnionitis→Antibiotics	1	0	NS
Fear, Desire for hospital	2	6	p 0.05
Desire for anesthesia→			
Anesthesia given	3	0	NS
Analgesia only	1	0	NS
Hyperemesis→IV's and Compazine	1	0	NS
Dropping FHT's			
No therapy, monitor applied	0	4	p 0.001
Cesarean section	0	1	NS
Cord prolapse→Cesarean	0	1	NS
With meconium→Intubation	0	3	p 0.025
Psychotic reaction to labor→Cesarean	0	1	NS

* sums of complications
† based on total N's (685 & 461 respectively)

TABLE 7 CONT'D
REASONS FOR TRANSPORTATION TO THE HOSPITAL & THERAPY APPLIED

COMPLICATION & THERAPY	M.D.'s N=58*	Midwives N=78*	Stat. Sign.†
2nd State Complications			
Protracted descent→			
Rx'ed with low forceps (1 FHT↓)	4	2	NS
Rx'ed with mid forceps with FHT↓	2	1	NS
Rx'ed with oxytocin	5	9	NS
Arrest			
CPD→Cesarean section	4	2	NS
Abnormal presentation→Mid forceps	1	1	NS
Brow presentation→Low forceps	0	1	NS
Dropping FHT's			
Low forceps	1	0	NS
With meconium→Oxytocin, intubation	0	2	NS
Mid forceps	1	0	NS
Bleeding→Oxytocin	0	1	NS
3rd Stage Complications			
Retained placenta→Manual removal	2	5	p<0.05
Hemorrhage→Oxytocin, Methergine, blood	1	4	p<0.025
Cervical laceration→Suturing	0	1	NS

* sums of complications
† based on total N's (685 & 461 respectively)

PERINATAL OUTCOME

Six sets of twins were successfully delivered at home, bringing the total number of births to 1,152. There was no maternal mortality or residual morbidity. Infant morbidity is summarized in Table 8 (p. 86).

Fifteen infants, including two sets of twins, weighed less than 2501 grams at birth. Eleven of these were over 2250 grams. Fourteen of the low birthweight infants were born at home.

One 1332 gram infant was born in the hospital following second trimester bleeding and remained there for a month. Two of the smaller babies weighing 1700 and 2200 grams were admitted to the hospital with mild respiratory distress syndrome. All the low birth weight babies survived without other postnatal complications than those mentioned above.

TABLE 8
INFANT MORBIDITY

Condition	Number	Rate per 1,000 LB	Delivery	Complications	Outcome
Congenital Defects	6	5.2			
PDA	1		Home	None	repaired surgically at 1 year
Coarctation of aorta	1		Home	None	repaired surgically at 2 years
Omphalocele	1		Home	None	repaired surgically at 15 hours
Myelomeningocele, thoracic	1		Home	None	mental & motor retardation at 18 mos.
Multiple minor anomalies	1		Hosp	FHT↓,c-s	no mental or motor retardation at 1 yr.
Down's syndrome	1		Home	Meconium	mental retardation
Cerebral Palsy	2	1.7			
Case one	1		Home	Meconium+++,FHT↓	motor retardation
Case two	1		Home	None	mild spastic with slow verbal develmnt.
Surgical Conditions	2	1.7	Home	None	pyloric stenosis repaired at 5 & 8 days
Low Birthweight	15	13.1			
Case one	1		Hosp	2nd Tri Bleed	1332 g, in hosp 1 mo., severe RDS
Case two	1		Home	None	1729 g, in hosp 2 wks., mild RDS
Case three	1		Home	Breech	2154 g, in hosp 12 days, mild RDS
Others	12		Home	None	No problems

As noted earlier, some mothers were medically screened out of the home delivery group because of premature labor. There were 20 such cases. If included, the total premature rate becomes 3.0%. (In California the prematurity rate in 1973 for white women, age 20-29, was 5.3%).

The average Apgar scores were 8.9 at 1 and 9.7 at 5 minutes, and were usually assessed by a nurse or lay midwife who did not deliver the infant. Forty infants (or 3.5%) born both at home and in the hospital had 1 minute Apgar scores of 4-6 and 7 infants (0.6%) had 1 minute Apgars of 3 or less and required resuscitation. (Drage and Berendes[5] have found a 21% incidence of 1 minute Apgar scores below 7.) Lack of drugs, both prenatally and intrapartum, may be associated with these relatively high scores.

Two other surviving infants were admitted to the hospital during the first 3 days; one for repair of an omphalocele, and one the result of the only unattended delivery with gross meconium staining and fetal distress, who was taken to the hospital within ten minutes after delivery, where intubation and lavage were not performed. This delivery was part of the lay midwife sample. Table 9 (below) describes the perinatal outcomes.

TABLE 9
PERINATAL OUTCOME

	Number	Study Rate	California Rate - 1973
Total Births*	1152		
Live Births*	1147		
Fetal Deaths	5	4.3†	10.2
Neonatal Deaths	6	5.2§	10.3
Total Perinatal Deaths	11	9.5†	20.3
Low Birthweight (<2501 g)	15	1.3%	6.4%

* Includes 6 sets of twins

† Fetal & perinatal death rates based on 1000 total births.

§ Neonatal death rates based on 1000 live births.

Four infants (or 0.3%) were neurologically abnormal at follow-up: 2 with cerebral palsy and 2 mentally retarded. This compares favorably to the 1.7% incidence of neurologically abnormal infants at 1 year found by the National Institute of Neurological Diseases and Stroke.[10] A fifth infant was slow, albeit consistent, in developing and did not walk until 18 months.

In addition to those listed in Table 9, there were 21 cases (or 1.8%) of jaundice requiring phototherapy. Only a few not already in the hospital were admitted, as parents were able to rig up fluorescent lights or, preferably, grow lights over bassinets at home.

Three cases of failure-to-thrive were switched from breast to bottle feeding with successful results. The average length of infant follow-up was 11.5 months. Some children are still being followed now at 3 to 5 years of age. Over 80% were followed at least 6 months.

The 9 women with previous fetal deaths had no complications.

Finally, the causes of fetal and infant deaths are given in Table 10 (p. 89). The perinatal mortality rate in this study is significantly lower than the 20.3 rate for the State of California in 1973. California's fetal death rate in 1973 for white women, age 20-29, was 8.2 per 1000 total births as compared to 4.3 in the home birth series. Unfortunately there is no comparable neonatal death rate available for this specific group.

There was no association in this series between length of first or second stage labor with the incidence of low Apgar scores at birth or other complications. Arrest of descent was weakly associated with somewhat lower Apgar scores, but this was also strongly associated with the use of forceps, and the total number of cases were too small to draw meaningful conclusions. There were 14 cases of prolonged rupture of membranes, but no resultant infections in the infants.

The average cost for home deliveries in the physician-directed services was $325 for mother and baby; for the entire study population, $277. This was an all inclusive rate, covering prenatal care, home visits postpartum and all necessary supplies. The average cost for total care with hospital delivery and 3 days' hospitalization was $1450. This latter figure is low as it does not include the additional fee for Cesarean section.

THE PLANNED HOSPITAL COMPARISON GROUP

The planned hospital comparison was drawn from the records of the Point Reyes family practice and consisted of 180 deliveries. These women came from the same population pool and had many of the same attitudinal sets as the women planning home delivery and would have been attended at home had they chosen this alternative. Women with complications of prenatal care obviating a home delivery who were delivered in the hospital were excluded from this sample.

For the hospital comparison group, 81.2% were followed at least six months. 129 of the infants and mothers were discharged at the end of two hours post-delivery. The hospital comparison group tended to be less from the counter-culture and were characterized by a more uniform middle class socioeconomic background with usually one or both parents a college graduate.

Table 11 (p. 90) compares the statistics on the selection of the study population. There were more primigravidae in the hospital group and fewer secundigravidae. The other differences were not significant. The maternal age was not statistically different between groups.

TABLE 10
CAUSES OF PERINATAL DEATH

Age at Death	Number	Delivery	Complications	Cause of Death
5 mos est gest age	1	Home	None	Rh incompatibility, insisted on home delivery
35 wks est gest age	2	Home	None	Intrauterine death, unknown cause
During labor	1	Hosp	Amnionitis IUD in place	Overwhelming intrauterine sepsis
During labor	1	Home	None	Unknown cause
2 days	1	Hosp	None	Macrosomia, single umbilical artery, bilateral adrenal hemorrhage, numerous congenital anomalies
7 days	1	Home	None	Cystic fibrosis, meconium ileus, postoperative peritonitis and sepsis
7 days	1	Home	None	Coarctation of aorta
10 days	1	Home	None	Cor biloculare
2 weeks	1	Home	None	Sudden infant death syndrome
3 weeks	1	Home	None	Post surgery for tetralogy of Fallot

TABLE 11
CHARACTERISTICS OF MOTHERS

| | Home | | Hosp | | Calif. | Stat. |
	Number	Percent	Number	Percent	1973	Sign.
Mother's Age	1146*	100.0%	180	100.0%	100.0%	NS
<20	60	5.2	12	6.7	17.3	NS
20-34	1068	93.2	160	89.9	77.6	NS
≥35	18	1.6	6	3.4	5.1	NS
Parity	1146	100.0%	180	100.0%	100.0%	
para 0	729	63.6	133	73.9	43.3	p<.005
para 1	237	20.7	33	18.3	31.0	NS
para 2	128	11.2	9	5.0	13.3	p<.025
para 3	34	3.0	2	1.1	6.0	NS
para 4	18	1.6	1	0.6	6.3	NS
Prentl Care Began	1146	100.0%	180	100.0%	100.0%	
1st Trimester	707	61.7	114	64.0	72.8	NS
2nd Trimester	362	31.6	63	35.4	20.2	NS
3rd Trimester	74	6.5	1	0.6	4.5	**
None	3	0.3	0	0.0	2.4†	NS

* For home group: Mean age=24.9, Range=16-44, Variance=16.8, SD=4.1
† Includes prenatal care unknown

Virtually all of the women in the planned hospital group were trained in childbirth classes (as were the home group) such as Bradley or Lamaze. A high incidence of breastfeeding also characterized the planned hospital group. All women in the planned hospital group attempted breastfeeding except for one. For a variety of reasons, two of these women were not successful.

RESULTS

Statistics on the presentations and deliveries are compared in Table 12 (p. 91). The planned hospital group contained more breech infants, had more Cesarean deliveries, had more analgesia, received more oxytocin during first, second, and after third stage labor, and had more low and mid forceps deliveries and episiotomies. It is important to note that their attendants had the same philosophies as the home delivery attendants, so that these differences come as a result of being in the hospital and may relate to a lower motivation for the women to have natural childbirth or to a more readily available analgesia or to a feeling of pressure transmitted to the birth attendants to intervene sooner and more aggressively in the hospital than in the home. These may all be related to the subtle effects of "atmosphere" which are, as yet, difficult to measure. The indications given for forceps and Cesarean deliveries are compared in Table 13 (p. 92). The planned hospital group had more Cesarean sections, primarily related to CPD and had more low forceps deliveries, significantly more because of a falling fetal heart rate.

TABLE 12
CHARACTERISTICS OF PRESENTATION & DELIVERY

	Home Number	Home Percent	Hosp Number	Hosp Percent	Statis. Signif.
Presentation	1146	100.0%	178	100.0%	
Vertex	1125	98.2	167	93.8	p<0.005
Brow	3	(0.3)	0	0.0	**
Shoulder	3	(0.3)	1	0.6	**
Breech	21	1.8	9	5.1	p<0.010
Delivery	1146	100.0%	178	100.0%	
Cesarean	28	2.4	10	5.6	p<0.025
Vaginal	1118	97.6	168	94.4	p<0.025
Analgesia only	14	(1.2)	9	(5.0)	p<0.025
Anesthesia only	3	(0.3)	3	(1.7)	**
Both	6	(0.5)	1	(0.6)	**
None	1095	(95.5)	154	(86.5)	p<0.001
Oxytocin					
1st & 2nd stage	85	7.4	29	15.3	p<0.001
3rd stage labor	235	20.5	54	30.3	p<0.005
Forceps					
Low forceps	11	1.0	7	3.9	p<0.001
Mid forceps	6	0.5	2	1.1	p<0.001
Perineal Lesions					
Laceratns req. repair	148	12.9	26	15.6	NS
Episiotomies	89	7.8	42	25.1	p<0.001

Table 14 (p. 93) presents the comparison complication figures for the planned hospital population, and compares these results with those obtained by the population delivering at home. The planned hospital group showed significantly more second stage labor dystocia (p<0.025), more drops of the fetal heart rate (p<0.005), more postpartum hemorrhage (p<0.001) and less "excessive bleeding" (defined as less than 650 ml. but more than the attendant is comfortable with) postpartum (p<0.001). The planned hospital population had significantly more forceps deliveries (p<0.001), episiotomies (p<0.001), Cesarean sections (p<0.025), and analgesia (p<0.001), and significantly less total unmedicated deliveries (p<0.001)

RELATIVE PERINATAL OUTCOME

Table 15 (p. 94) compares the perinatal outcome data. The neonatal mortality and perinatal mortality results were not significantly different between the planned hospital group and the home delivery group, nor was the rate of low birthweight infants, or the mean length of infant follow-up. The hospital neonatal death rate was 5.5 per 1000 with 11.1 perinatal deaths per 1000.

TABLE 13
INDICATIONS FOR C-SECTIONS AND FORCEPS DELIVERIES
IN WOMEN BEGINNING LABOR AT HOME

	Home Number	Hosp Number
Low Forceps Delivery		
Protracted descent	6	0
Arrest of descent	2	3
Dysfunctional labor	1	0
Brow presentation with arrest of descent	1	0
Fetal heart drop	1	3
Bleeding during 2nd stage	0 ―― 11	1 ―― 7
Mid Forceps Delivery		
Protracted descent	3	0
Arrest of descent	1	1
Dysfunctional labor	1	0
Fetal heart drop, occiput posterior (OP) pres.	1	0
FHT↓, amnionitis, maternal hypertension	0 ―― 6	1 ―― 2
C-Sections		
Cephalopelvic disproportion (CPD)	16	7
Failure to descend, OP presentation, rel. CPD	6	0
Arrest of active dilation, FHT↓, cord 4x neck	1	0
Prolapsed cord	1	(1)
Breech with amnionitis	1	0
Psychotic reaction to labor	1	0
Acutely dropping fetal heart tones	1	0
Toxemia	1	0
Breech with low breech score, poor labor progress	0	1
Transverse lie with one prolapsed cord	(1) ―― 28	2 ―― 10

TABLE 14
COMPLICATIONS OF LABOR & DELIVERY (HOSPITAL GROUP)
(INDIVIDUAL WOMEN MAY BE LISTED UNDER MORE THAN 1 COMPLICATION)

PRIMIGRAVIDAE (N=52/133=39.1%)				MULTIGRAVIDAE (N=10/45=22.2%)			
Complication	Hosp	Percent	Statis. Sign.[†]	Complication	Hosp	Percent	Statis. Sign.[†]
Intrapartum				Intrapartum			
Dystocia[2] 1st stage	15	11.3	NS	Dystocia[2] 1st stage	2	4.4	NS
Dystocia 2nd stage	10	7.5	p<0.025	Dystocia 2nd stage	1	2.2	NS
CPD	7	5.3	NS	CPD with breech	1	2.2	--
Meconium stain only	4	3.0	NS	Precipitous labor	2	4.4	NS
FHT↓(c̄,s̄ meconium)	10	7.5	p<0.005	FHT↓	1	2.2	NS
Hypertension	2	1.5	NS	Hypertension	1	2.2	--
Precipitous labor	2	1.5	NS	Transverse lie	1	2.2	--
Other*	6	4.5	--	TOTAL	9		
TOTAL	56						
Postpartum				Postpartum			
Hemorrhage[3]	5	3.8	p<0.001	Hemorrhage[3]	0	--	NS
Excessive PP bleeding[3]	2	1.5	p<0.001	Excessive PP bleeding[3]	1	2.2	NS
Retained placenta	2	1.5	NS	Retained placenta	1	2.2	NS
Endometritis	3	2.3	NS	Endometritis	1	2.2	NS
PP Depression	1	0.8	NS	TOTAL	3		
TOTAL	13						

* single cases of amnionitis, shoulder presentation, cord prolapse, cord knot, recurrent pyelonephritis, transverse lie.
† compared with Table 5 on page 81.

1 Percent complications per 133 primigravidae, 45 multigravidae.
2 Dystocia as used in this table is defined as prolonged or arrested 1st stage, failure to dilate; prolonged or arrested 2nd stage, failure to descend, according to Friedman & Greenhill (1974).
3 Hemorrhage is defined as more than 650 ml; excessive bleeding as "more than normal", and includes late bleeding after the 3rd postpartum day.

TABLE 15
COMPARATIVE PERINATAL OUTCOME

	Home Number	Rate	Hosp Number	Rate	Calif. 1973	Stat. Sign.
Total Births	1152*		180†			
Live Births	1147*		180†			
Fetal Deaths	5	4.3α	1	5.5α	8.2α,γ	NS
Neonatal Deaths	6	5.2β	1	5.5β	10.3β	NS
Total Perinatal Deaths	11	9.5γ	2	11.1α	20.3α	NS
Low Birthweight (<2501 g)	15	1.3β	3	1.7β	5.3β,γ	NS
Mean Length of Infant Follow-up	11.5 mos.		11.6 mos.			NS
S.D. Length of Follow-up	10.3 mos.		10.4 mos			NS
% Infants Followd to 6 mos.	83.4%		81.2%			NS

* includes 6 sets of twins.
† includes 2 sets of twins.

α 1 per 1000 total births
β 1 per 1000 live births
γ for white, non-Spanish surname, age 20-29

Table 16 (p. 95) presents infant morbidity for the hospital group. Table 17 (pp. 96-97) compares neonatal complications. The planned hospital group had significantly more fetal hypoxia (p<0.025) and significantly more 1 minute Apgar scores less than 4 (p<0.025). Among the homebirth series, the midwives had more infants who received phototherapy for jaundice than did the physicians (p<0.025). Causes of fetal deaths are compared in Table 18 (p. 98).

The prematurity rate for the population initially seeking assistance from one of the services studied was 3.0%. For the planned hospital population it was 2.8%. There was no significant differences between 1 minute Apgar scores ranging from 4-6 between the homebirth group and the planned hospital group with 40 & 7 such ratings, respectively. Average Apgar scores for the planned hospital group were 8.6 at 1 minute and 9.7 which were not significantly different from the homebirth group.

There was no association among the hospital group either between length of labor and length of second stage of incidence of low Apgar scores at birth or other complications.

TABLE 16
INFANT MORBIDITY OF PLANNED HOSPITAL GROUP*

Complication	Number	Rate per 1,000 LB	Delivery	Complications	Outcome
Low Birthweight	3	16.6	Hosp		
Case one	1		Hosp	FHT↓ prior to del.	neonatal sepsis and amnionitis
Case two	1		Hosp	None	mild RDS
Case three	1		Hosp	None	mild RDS
Hyperviscosity syndrome	1	5.5	Hosp	None	resolved

* To compare these data with the homebirth group, see Table 8, p. 86.

The mean length of 1st stage labor among the group planning hospital birth was 12.5 hrs for primigravidae and 5.4 hrs for multigravidae. For the home group it was 10.2 hrs and 4.6 hrs respectively. The standard deviations were 2.6 and 1.3 hrs, respectively, for planned hospital group and 1.9 and 1.2 hrs, respectively, for planned home group. This difference was significant at $p < 0.05$.

The mean length of 2nd stage labor for the planned hospital primigravidae was 106.8 min ± 31.0 min and for multigravidae was 50.1 min ± 28.3 min. For the home series, the mean length of 2nd stage was 118.2 min ± 40.5 min for primigravidae and 44.6 min ± 23.7 min for multigravidae. The primigravidae differences were significant at $p < 0.05$. Multigravidae were not comparable for parity and could not be compared.

There were 14 cases of prolonged rupture of membranes in the homebirth series and 11 in the planned hospital series ($p < 0.01$). There were no infections of the infants except for one low birthweight infant whose mother developed amnionitis. She was in the planned hospital series.

TABLE 17
COMPARATIVE NEONATAL OUTCOMES

| COMPLICATIONS | HOME PRIMIGRAVIDAE N=729 | | | | STATIS. SIGNIF.[1] |
| | M.D.'s N=464 | | Midwives N=265 | | |
	Home	To Hosp	Home	To Hosp	
Jaundice Req. Rx	1	5	2	9	p<0.025
Fetal Hypoxia	2	0	0	0	NS
Neurological Abnormalities[2,3]	2	1	0	1	NS
Cerebral Palsy	1	0	0	1	NS
Neonatal FTT	1	1	0	1	NS
Apgar (1 min.) Score < 4	3	0	1	1	NS
Score = 4-6	12	7	5	3	NS

| COMPLICATIONS | HOME MULTIGRAVIDAE N=417 | | | | STATIS. SIGNIF.[1] |
| | M.D.'s N=221 | | Midwives N=196 | | |
	Home	To Hosp	Home	To Hosp	
Jaundice Req. Rx	2	1	0	1	NS
Fetal Hypoxia	0	1	0	0	NS
Neurological Abnormalities[2,3]	0	0	0	1	NS
Cerebral Palsy	0	0	0	0	NS
Neonatal FTT	0	0	0	0	NS
Apgar (1 min.) Score < 4	0	1	0	1	NS
Score = 4-6	2	4	2	5	NS

| COMPLICATIONS | HOME TOTAL N=1146 | | | | STATIS. SIGNIF.[1] |
| | M.D.'s N=685 | | Midwives N=461 | | |
	Home	To Hosp	Home	To Hosp	
Jaundice Req. Rx	3	6	2	10	p<0.025
Fetal Hypoxia	2	1	0	0	NS
Neurological Abnormalities[2,3]	2	1	0	2	NS
Cerebral Palsy	1	0	0	1	NS
Neonatal FTT	1	1	0	1	NS
Apgar (1 min.) Score < 4	3	1	1	2	NS
Score = 4-6	14	11	7	8	NS

Cont'd on next page

TABLE 17 CONT'D
COMPARATIVE NEONATAL OUTCOMES

COMPLICATIONS	PLANNED	STATIS. SIGNIF.[1]
Jaundice Req. Rx	3	NS
Fetal Hypoxia	3	p<0.025
Neurological Abnormalities[2,3]	0	NS
Cerebral Palsy	0	NS
Neonatal FTT	1	NS
Apgar (1 min.) Score < 4	6	p<0.025
Score = 4-6	7	NS

[1] Calculated on the basis of home & hospital
[2] Includes cerebral palsied infants
[3] Development at 1 year follow-up

CONCLUSION

In conclusion, the home delivery group of women were a self-selected group screened for obvious problems and complications occurring during pregnancy, while the hospital group is a similarly selected group who would have been eligible for a home delivery had they decided to have one. While the home delivery outcomes are not directly comparable to State statistics, their outcomes are better than average and lower than might have been expected. Behrman et al.[2] have studied 39,000 white middle-class women in Oregon receiving prenatal care from private physicians and found a neonatal mortality rate of 12 per 1000 live births and a perinatal mortality rate of 17 per 1000 total births. Interestingly enough, if one eliminated premature infants from Behrman's series, the neonatal death rate was 5.5 per 1000 and the perinatal death rate was 7.5 per 1000 which is not statistically significantly different from the home delivery series of this report (cf. Table 15, p. 94).

Another often asked question is that of the need for routine fetal monitoring. Chan et al.[4] have studied the role of fetal monitoring in reducing intrapartum deaths, and in a study in which patients were randomly assigned to fetal monitoring, there was no statistically significant difference between the monitored group and the non-monitored group. Also important is that Chan's study revealed an intrapartum death rate of 1.7 per 1000 in his 1162 monitored patients. This is not statistically significantly different from the intrapartum death rate of 0.95 per 1000 in our series of 1146 home deliveries. In another study, Shenker et al.[13] reported a 0.5 per 1000 intrapartum death rate in monitored patients. This is not statistically significantly different from our series either.

TABLE 18
CAUSES OF PERINATAL DEATH IN PLANNED HOSPITAL GROUP*

Age At Death	Number	Delivery	Complications	Cause of Death
During labor	1	Hosp	Rapidly ↓ FHT	Meningoencephalitis, etiology unknown
8 days	1	Hosp	None	Aplastic left ventricle

* To compare these data with the homebirth group, see Table 10, p. 89

Shenker et al.[13] did, however, show a significant decrease in intrapartum deaths in the monitored series versus the unmonitored series in Bellevue Hospital in New York City. Clearly, the nursing care in Bellevue Hospital is not adequate, which brings us to recent studies from the West Coast showing an equivalent success rate of nurses versus fetal monitor, but with less infections reported with the nurses. It is not hard to imagine which was the more supportive personal care.

Other important points can be made. The perineal massage technique used by the midwives to aid in preventing vaginal lacerations during delivery was effective, and, as the physicians adopted this technique, their laceration rate decreased. The higher utilization of oxytocin after delivery by the physicians may have reflected its availability to them and their training to use it frequently. The equivalence of hemorrhage and blood loss results between the physician and midwife group suggests that it was not needed as frequently as used. The lay midwives took women to the hospital more frequently than the physicians, presumably reflecting their decreased capabilities to handle specific complications at home and their lower threshold level for going to the hospital possibly related to a lower level of knowledge. The physicians were able to treat some of their cases of uterine inertia with buccal oxytocin at home, and removed several retained placenta at home, as well as carrying oxytocin and Methergine to treat third stage bleeding at home. The greater number of FHT problems brought to the hospital by the midwives may reflect their greater level of anxiety in dealing with and desire for transporting abnormal situations to the hospital early.

Comparisons with the planned hospital group suggest that for women delivering at home with the philosophies and practices of this particular group of practitioners, there was no significant increase in risk with a home delivery versus a hospital delivery. In fact, by avoidance of obstetrical medication, such as was used more frequently in the hospital by equivalently prepared women (presumably because of the effect of the hospital atmosphere on the encouragement for obstetrical medication), the incidence of low Apgar scores was less at home than was the incidence of fetal hypoxia.

The greater use of analgesia in labor by the planned hospital group may have also contributed to their greater incidence of second stage dystocia and greater incidence of fetal heart rate drops. The breech infants did not contribute to these problems. The incidence of postpartum hemorrhage was greater in the planned hospital group and may represent the greater tendency to pull on the umbilical cord to aid in the delivery of the placenta. At home, the umbilical cord was rarely pulled to aid placental delivery, but rather, the natural expulsive forces of the uterus were relied upon. This is substantiated by the longer third stages seen in the home group. The contribution of other factors such as lower stress in the home environment, alternative delivery positions, and the like cannot be assessed in a study such as this, but may be significant.

Of note, as well, are the close similarity of these findings to the home delivery statistics in the Netherlands (personal communication, Jan Kloosterman, MD, University of Amsterdam) and to home delivery statistics compiled by Gregory White, MD,[15] in Chicago, and by Victor Berman, MD,[3] in Los Angeles.

Generally, the response of physicians to home delivery has been negative. Many view homebirth as an irresponsible risk to mother and child. They do not encourage or attend home deliveries, and many have refused to give prenatal care, advice, or instruction to couples planning homebirth. A dichotomy exists in obstetrics today between the technological trend represented by high risk obstetric units with fetal monitoring and readily available medical and surgical intervention, and the family-centered, natural childbirth trend represented in its extreme by couples planning home delivery *without medical support*. We feel that reducing the antagonism between these divergent poles would enhance care for women choosing hospital as well as home deliveries.

More studies of this kind are needed before any conclusions can be drawn. We are currently engaged in a study in which we are attempting to match a comparison hospital group. However, evidence from this study population already strongly suggests that home delivery is a safe alternative for medically screened healthy women; they deserve adequate care for the delivery of their choice. This would include prenatal care by a physician, childbirth education, and only necessary intervention by attendants. Hospitals should be encouraged to adopt those techniques of homebirth that improve pregnancy outcome, which might include perineal massage and gentle head delivery to avoid episiotomies and lacerations, choice of the use of analgesia and anesthesia, and generally provide a supportive, friendly, and comfortable environment for labor and delivery.

Finally, what these statistics have missed is the importance of the spiritual and the emotional aspects of birth. Someday, perhaps, we will be able to empirically validate what our feelings tell us is true.

REFERENCES

1. Aaro, L.A., Saed, F: Low-incidence Cesarean Section: 12-year experience. Mayo Clinic Proc. 50:365-369, 1975.

2. Behrman, R.E., Babson, G.S., and Lessel, R.: Fetal and Neonatal Mortality in White Middle Class Infants. Am. J. Dis. Child 121:486-489, 1971.

3. Berman, V: Comment at First Annual Meeting of the North American Society of Psychosomatic Obstetrics and Gynecology (NASPOG) Chicago, Illinois, April 10, 1976.

4. Chan, W.H., Paul, R.H., and Toews, J.: Intrapartum Fetal Monitoring. Ob.Gyn.41:7-13, 1973.

5. Drage, J.S., Berendes, H: Apgar Scores and Outcome of the Newborn. Pediat. Clin. N. Amer. 13:635-643, 1966.

6. Eastman, N.J., Hellman, L.M.: Williams Obstetrics. New York, Appleton-Century-Crofts, 1966, p. 988

7. Friedman, E.A.: Patterns of Labor as Indicators of Risk. Clin. Ob.Gyn.16:172-183, 1973.

8. Hazell, L.D.: A Study of 300 Elective Home Births. Birth & the Family Jour. 2:11-18, 1975.

9. Klaus, M., Fanaroff, A.: Care of the High Risk Neonate. Toronto, Wm Saunders Co., 1973, p. 141

10. Lang, R.: The Birth Book. Ben Lomond, California, Genesis Press, 1972.

11. Mehl, L.E., Peterson, G.H., White, M.C., and Hayes, W.: Outcomes of Elective Home Births: A Series of 1146 Cases. Paper presented at the First Annual Meeting of the North American Society for Psychosomatic Obstetrics and Gynecology, Chicago, April 10, 1976.

12. Niswander, K.R., Gordon, M.: The Women and Their Pregnancies. The Collaborative Perinatal Study of the National Institute of Neurological Diseases and Stroke. U.S. Dept. HEW, Philadelphia, W.B. Saunders Co., 1972, p. 49

13. Shenker, L., Post, R.C., Seiler, J.S.: Routine Electronic Monitoring of the Fetal Heart Rate and Uterine Activity During Labor. Ob.Gyn.46:185-189, 1975.

14. State of California, Department of Health, Center for Health Statistics, 1975.

15. White, G.: Home and Hospital Delivery, 25 Years Experience With Each. Paper presented at the First Annual Meeting of NASPOG, Chicago, April 10, 1976.

PERINATAL AND MATERNAL MORTALITY RATES BY TYPE OF HOSPITAL

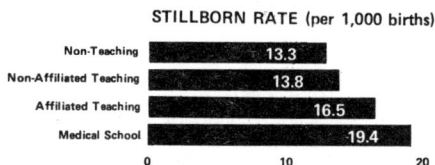

STILLBORN RATE (per 1,000 births)

Non-Teaching	13.3
Non-Affiliated Teaching	13.8
Affiliated Teaching	16.5
Medical School	19.4

0   10   20

Prepared By:

Doris B. Haire, DMS, President
American Foundation for
        Maternal & Child Health
30 Beekman Place
New York, NY 10022

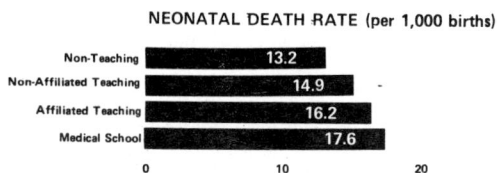

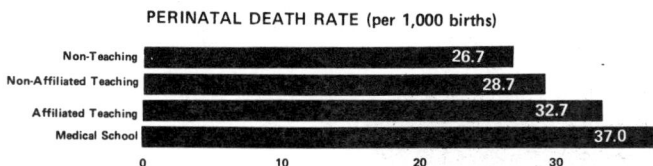

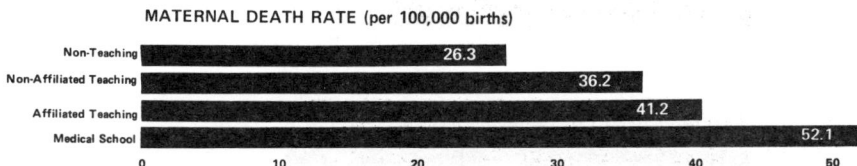

NEONATAL DEATH RATE (per 1,000 births)

Non-Teaching	13.2
Non-Affiliated Teaching	14.9
Affiliated Teaching	16.2
Medical School	17.6

0   10   20

PERINATAL DEATH RATE (per 1,000 births)

Non-Teaching	26.7
Non-Affiliated Teaching	28.7
Affiliated Teaching	32.7
Medical School	37.0

0   10   20   30

MATERNAL DEATH RATE (per 100,000 births)

Non-Teaching	26.3
Non-Affiliated Teaching	36.2
Affiliated Teaching	41.2
Medical School	52.1

0   10   20   30   40   50

DEFINITIONS:
Stillborn—Fetus weighing 500 grams or more and born dead.
Neonatal Death—Death of a liveborn infant within the first
        28 days of life.
Perinatal Death—Stillbirths plus Neonatal Deaths.

SOURCE:
National Study of Maternity Care: Survey of Obstetric Practice and Associated Services in Hospitals in the United States
by the Committee on Maternal Health of the American College
of Obstetricians and Gynecologists, 1970.

PERINATAL AND MATERNAL MORTALITY RATES BY SIZE OF HOSPITAL

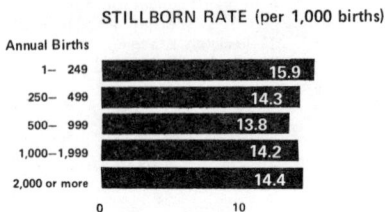

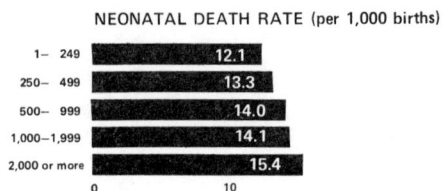

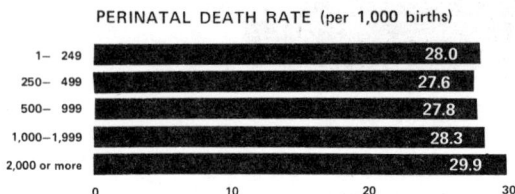

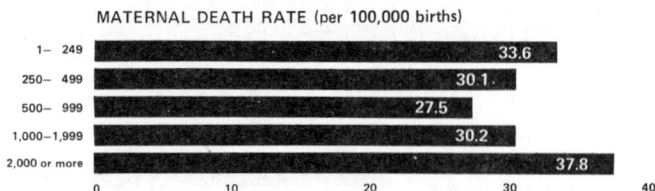

STILLBORN RATE (per 1,000 births)

Annual Births

1– 249	15.9
250– 499	14.3
500– 999	13.8
1,000–1,999	14.2
2,000 or more	14.4

0   10

While the public is being advised by various health agencies of the need to eliminate small and medium-sized obstetric services, a national survey by the American College of Obstetricians and Gynecologists reveals that, in general (and particularly in hospitals with 500 or more annual births), the larger obstetric services tend to have a greater rate of maternal and infant deaths. The ACOG study also showed that the stronger the affiliation between the obstetric service and a medical school the greater the rate of maternal and infant deaths. Undoubtedly some of these deaths result from the fact that there is a greater rate of high-risk mothers in larger teaching hospitals, but it is also likely that the greater tendency to intervene in the normal progress of labor and birth in these institutions, especially in order to provide learning opportunities for students and residents, contributes to the poorer maternal and infant outcome in these institutions and may also result in a disproportinately high incidence of neurologically damaged children.

NEONATAL DEATH RATE (per 1,000 births)

1– 249	12.1
250– 499	13.3
500– 999	14.0
1,000–1,999	14.1
2,000 or more	15.4

0   10

PERINATAL DEATH RATE (per 1,000 births)

1– 249	28.0
250– 499	27.6
500– 999	27.8
1,000–1,999	28.3
2,000 or more	29.9

0   10   20   30

MATERNAL DEATH RATE (per 100,000 births)

1– 249	33.6
250– 499	30.1
500– 999	27.5
1,000–1,999	30.2
2,000 or more	37.8

0   10   20   30   40

DEFINITIONS:
Stillborn—Fetus weighing 500 grams or more and born dead.
Neonatal Death—Death of a liveborn infant within the first
    28 days of life.
Perinatal Death—Stillbirths plus Neonatal Deaths.

SOURCE:
National Study of Maternity Care: Survey of Obstetric Practice and Associated Services in Hospitals in the United States by the Committee on Maternal Health of the American College of Obstetricians and Gynecologists, 1970.

A Safe Homebirth Program That Works

Janet L. Epstein, RN, CNM
Marion F. McCartney, RN, CNM
James D. Brew, Jr., MD, FACOG
& Ludovic J. DeVocht, MD, FACOG

INTRODUCTION
(James Brew)

My relationships to nurse midwives have been stretched over a period of time from 1956, with Certified Nurse Midwives, and since 1974, with Registered Nurse Midwives--because they have only recently begun registration in the three jurisdictions of this area: viz., Maryland, Virginia, and the District of Columbia.

The critics of "homebirth services" are a motley group. They include people both for and against homebirth. There's the OB-GYN News, the American College of Obstetricians and Gynecologists, and the American College of Nurse Midwives. But they are even more general than that--like the Washington Post, Redbook Magazine, Cosmopolitan, the Ladies Home Journal, and more. It just depends on what you read. You can find arguments both for and against home delivery and for and against nurse midwives, but I just want to say that I am completely in favor of nurse midwifery so whatever I say here is completely biased and I am not likely to give a two-sided story in any respect.

---

* JANET EPSTEIN is President of the Maternity Center Associates, a working homebirth service that began in October, 1975, in the Washington, DC, Area with Headquarters in Bethesda, Maryland; She is a member of the American College of Nurse Midwives and the Nurses Association of the American College of OB-GYN.

* MARION McCARTNEY is Vice President of the Maternity Center Associates; and is a member of the American College of Nurse Midwives and the Nurses Association of the American College of OB-GYN.

* JAMES BREW, JR, is on the Staff of the Maternity Center Associates; a faculty member of Georgetown Medical College; Senior Attending Obstetrician at Washington Hospital Center, former Chief OB-GYN, District of Columbia General Hospital; a Fellow of the American College of Obstetricians & Gynecologists and a Fellow of the American College of Surgeons.

* LUDOVIC DeVOCHT is on the Staff of the Maternity Center Associates; and was formerly at Coth University of Levoin, Belgium, & Lariboisiere Hospital, Paris, France. He was scheduled to speak at the NAPSAC Conference with the other participants of the M.C.A. but could not come at the last moment because of the progressing labor of one of the mothers under his care.

I am a member of the Committee of the District of Columbia Medical Society for Maternity Welfare. I am sort of a maverick. They keep me on the committee because they want to hear how the rest of the world lives. I am the only one on the Committee who does home deliveries. Last year they spent one whole meeting, which is 1/10 of all their meetings for the year, on what to do with people who deliver babies at home. And then, this year, thay have already spent two meetings on what to do about nurse midwives. So it is not all calm and I sit in the middle of it--sometimes in a defensive posture and sometimes in a posture that is helpful to the cause. Nevertheless it is supposed to be a method of keeping communications going--whatever communications mean, because sometimes they don't mean a thing.

The most important thing I wish to say about the Maternity Center Associates here in this area is that it is a group that has a program that works. I hope we can make you understand that it works because so many people, including doctors and non-doctors, can't believe that such a situation can work.

One of the reasons it does work is that certain freedoms of authority have been delegated by Dr. DeVocht and myself to the discretion of the nurse midwives. These we call our "standing orders" and are specified in writing and in detail (see pp.112-114) for a complete listing of these). If you are going to make something work you have to be able to put it down in black and white so people can really see it. This group has put all the procedures down in such a way that even though I had been practicing home deliveries for 18 years and had loosely put together rules of what I would do, would not do, and so on, I had never actually put it all in one nice folder in a few pages as they have done (all of this material is published here on pp. 107-122). The standing orders enable the nurse midwives to order and prescribe things that, usually, only doctors can do. It is a list of things the nurse midwives are permitted to do, and are supposed to do, on their own initiative in the cases that they treat.

Now I won't go into the complete listing of these here because they are printed in their entirety later (pp. 112-114) but let me briefly go over a few items. For example, they may write orders for Bendectin, ferrous fumarate, folic acid, and multivitamins. Now, all of these things are not necessarily prescription items. Some are over-the-counter. Douches, for example, are all over-the-counter. Laxatives are over-the-counter except Lomotil which they can prescribe. After long discussion, we also decided on two main antibiotics which they can prescribe without consultation: Gantrisin or AZO for urinary tract infections and ampicillin for breast infections. Xylocaine is permitted for repair of episiotomies and Pitocin is allowed postpartum.

They also get into family planning which includes prescription of oral contraceptives, the fitting, introduction and use of IUDs, diaphragms and, of course, the discussion of other items like foam, condoms, rhythm, and basal temperature. All the ordinary laboratory examinations, likewise, may be ordered. This is handled specifically by using the names of the physicians who act as "backups."

The need for medical "backup" can be a problem. For one thing, it is not always clear what is implied by "backup." Nevertheless, Dr. DeVocht and I are members of the Maternity Center Associates and, as such, are "full time backups" for these midwives. We will go to the hospital or to the home as appropriate to the situation. In addition to us, there are also 8 other cooperative physicians distributed through the area who will give hospital admittance when necessary and, in this sense, also serve as "backups." In this way, the Maternity Center Associates has access to a number of area hospitals so that as the need arises one of the nearer hospitals can be approached.

BRIEF DESCRIPTION OF THE MCA HOMEBIRTH SERVICE
(Janet Epstein)

We have a very active and growing homebirth service here in the Washington Metropolitan Area and it is incorporated. One of the reasons it is incorporated is that the State of Maryland specifies that nurse midwives may not practice independently nor collect a direct fee for their services. So, in order to get around that, we incorporated and, therefore, it is the Corporation that collects the fee for the services, not us personally. We then derive a salary from the Corporation which, I am pleased to say, we can do from our service. There are three nurse midwives working with MCA right now actively. Two of the nurse midwives own the Corporation and one is an employee of the Corporation. Our administrative set-up is simple and straight forward. One thing we cannot do, as yet, is to collect third party payment from Blue Cross-Blue Shield. However, some of the other agencies will pay nurse midwives--for instance, Etna, Government Etna, and some of the small union insurance companies. We feel we are making some headway in terms of this sort of recognition and expect more such companies will agree to pay for our services in the future.

Our services include caring for *normal* women and their families. I want to stress the term, *normal*, because as a nurse midwife, or as a nurse in general, I believe that our unique function is that of caring for normal, healthy people. There are physicians and some kinds of nurses who are very concerned with unhealthy people and I think this is also very important. But I think that the healthy lady, or the healthy "anybody" for that matter, can sometimes be thrown aside and neglected. So we believe that our unique goal is with the healthy women. Therefore, we do not call our women "patients." We call them "clients" because they are healthy people who have just come to us for advice and assistance. If we do find a "client" who is not healthy, we try to refer her to an appropriate physician who can take care of her, or if she already has someone in mind to whom she would rather go, that is fine also.

WE DON'T CALL OUR WOMEN "PATIENTS." WE CALL THEM "CLIENTS" BECAUSE THEY ARE HEALTHY PEOPLE WHO HAVE JUST COME TO US FOR ADVICE AND ASSISTANCE. IF WE DO FIND A "CLIENT" WHO IS NOT HEALTHY, WE REFER HER TO AN APPROPRIATE PHYSICIAN.

We have a lot of screening criteria (described in full on pp. 108-110). We are very, very careful whom we select for homebirth. We also maintain a lot of regulation concerning the management of our program in order to insure the ultimate goal of safety in homebirth for the individual.

Somebody made the statement that if women want homebirths, the professionals providing women prenatal care would have to practice improved, if not superior, prenatal care. I think that is absolutely true. We see our clients, as usual, as an obstetrician would--usually once a month until they are about 28 weeks pregnant or more often if indicated, twice a month until they are 36 weeks pregnant, and then weekly, if they desire, until they deliver.

One thing we try to offer at MCA is a lot of options.   Insofar as the situation remains normal, our clients can do and suggest almost anything. We have had clients want to use a variety of different positions in labor, want to handle their babies in particular ways. So long as we see that things remain normal, we are very broad. We will use some of Leboyer's methods--as much or as little as the individual wants. We will turn out lights, turn on lights, bathe, not bathe. It really doesn't matter to us. We consider ourselves just as hired experts only there to help and to monitor things so that everything goes well.

We usually try to make one visit to the client's home before she goes into labor just so that we will know how to get there at 3:00 in the morning when it is snowing a blizzard outside. Also, we try to establish a very warm, friendly, close relationship so that we are always on a first name basis. We don't wear uniforms. When the woman is in labor, we have a shirt that Marion and I wear that says on it, *"THE HAPPY BABY HOME DELIVERY SERVICE."* We wear that shirt with blue jeans which helps to keep things casual and optimistic.

We ask each client to hire or secure another nurse or professional who knows how to do some minimal nursing procedures and who can act as a birth assistant. In this way, each birth is attended by both an experienced midwife and a birth assistant. We usually come to the home once labor has been reasonably well established. From there we just sort of coast along, watching, and as long as everything remains normal, we complete the delivery at home. We do not do anything routine at home, which includes such things as shaves, enemas, episiotomies, or anything like that. Such things are done only "as needed."

WE TRY TO ESTABLISH A VERY WARM, FRIENDLY, CLOSE RELATIONSHIP SO THAT WE ARE ALWAYS ON A FIRST NAME BASIS. WE DON'T WEAR UNIFORMS. INSTEAD WE WEAR BLUE JEANS WITH SHIRTS THAT SAY "HAPPY BABY HOME DELIVERY SERVICE" WHICH HELPS TO KEEP THINGS CASUAL AND OPTIMISTIC.

During the immediate postpartum, we stay with the mother usually about 2 hours. We do administer silver nitrate since it is a
State Law here in Maryland (our client information sheet on silver
nitrate is given on p. 122). Aquamephyton is optional, depending on
whether the mother or the baby's physician wants it. The women select a pediatrician who agrees to come to their home within 24 hours.
Most of the pediatricians here have been very cooperative about that.

Regarding finances, we charge our clients $450. This includes
all prenatal care, prenatal visits to the home, labor, and delivery
at home, as well as postpartum care and a postpartum visit. The postpartum care includes a 2 week check-up, a 6 week check-up, a 6 month
check-up, and a one year check-up. We also have postpartum groups
run by a psychiatric nurse practitioner who sees our clients for 3
group sessions. These are at no additional cost to the client, being
included in our $450 fee. The emphasis there is, of course, on new
family relationships and the crisis that can occur by having a new
baby in the family. The only extra charges that might happen would
be for extra blood work or laboratory tests. If for some reason the
client needs to be seen by a physician, we usually refund part of her
fee so that the total amount she spends still remains close to the
original $450.

Our malpractice insurance as nurse midwives is for $200-600,000
coverage and we only pay $15 per year for it. It is very, very low
because, so far, nurse midwives have not been sued. As soon as one
of us gets sued, it will go up accordingly. One thing that we do
that helps to minimize the tendency for suit is to freely inform the
client of what we are doing and its limitations so that she offers
her *informed* consent--thus sharing the responsibility. For example,
if asked about the safety of the medications we may use, we honestly
answer that "none of the drugs we are giving has been proven safe."
So that is another reason our malpractice may be low. Another thing,
of course, is that we have Dr. Brew and Dr. DeVocht to back us up.
Dr. Brew's insurance premium is something like $5,500 a year but is
no higher than any other hospital-based obstetrician. Being a homebirth physician does not, in itself, increase the risk of malpractice
in the eyes of insurance companies. Ultimately, Dr. Brew and Dr. De-
Vocht are responsible for what Marion and I do. If we really mess up
sometime, they will probably get sued along with us. So they are
really sticking their necks out for us.

MCA SCREENING CRITERIA & STATISTICS
(Marion McCartney)

As part of our home delivery service we decided when we started
out that we would run a research project to test our screening criteria. Our screening criteria are pretty much the same as any other
nurse midwifery service in that we are taking medically uncomplicated
women--women who have a normal pregnancy and a normal labor and
delivery (a complete list of MCA screening criteria is given on pp.
108-110). What we are trying to do is to show that these screening
criteria can successfully screen out a low risk population. This has
significance for any out-of-hospital service. You really want to find
who your low risk mothers are. Our screening criteria are explained
to the client as she enters the service.

ABOUT HALF OF OUR CLIENTS ARE DELIVERED BY THE BABY'S FATHER RATHER THAN BY THE NURSE MIDWIFE. WE HAVE TAUGHT PEOPLE WHO HAVE NEVER SEEN A DELIVERY HOW TO DELIVER A LADY OVER AN INTACT PERINEUM. IT REALLY CAN BE DONE VERY EASILY.

So far, we have done 71 deliveries in the first seven months of our service, and the practice has been increasing as we have gone along. We started with two midwives and now have three. We were turning people away. We now can handle about 20 births a month.

Out of those 71 deliveries we have had 37 primigravidae and 32 who were multiparous--so our service has been about half and half. Out of this group we have hospitalized 14 people (or 20%). Of these 14 who needed hospitalization, 2 were multiparous and 12 (or 86%) were primagravidae . One of the multiparous mothers had a Cesarean section because she was in premature labor and the fetus was in distress when she got into the hospital. The other multipara had prolonged rupture of membranes with meconium but did deliver spontaneously. Among the 12 primigravidae , the most significant thing was that 5 of them had unengaged heads after they had been in labor for 3 or 4 hours. Of that group, 4 had Cesarean sections and one delivered spontaneously. Of the remaining 7 hospitalized primigravidae , 2 experienced fetal distress of which one was delivered by forceps and the other spontaneously. Another showed meconium when the membranes ruptured; the baby came spontaneously but had respiratory distress. Another simply had prolonged rupture of membranes but delivered spontaneously. The last 3 had prolonged 2nd stage: 1 delivered spontaneously and 2 required outlet forceps. We have so far had no mortality and no morbidity.

I think that the few statistics we have already is a reflection of what is going to happen over the next few years. We will eventually be publishing a greater survey for a larger number of people so that we can really show something significant about what we are doing. I think that our statistics will say that you can, in fact, screen out high risk and select low risk for treatment in a facility which is more in tune with her healthy state rather than treating her as if she were at death's door and needed all the medical equipment required only for high risk obstetrics.

Dr. Brew's experience has already shown that adequate screening can be done. Two years ago, he did an analysis of the 489 home deliveries he had done up to that time and only had 3 postpartum hemorrhages in 489 births of which only 1 had to be transfused. On a random basis you ordinarily have to expect about 4% postpartum hemorrhages so that he should have had somewhere in the neighborhood of 19 or 20 postpartum hemorrhages. This result means that the 489 were a very select group of mothers. In the 71 cases so far treated by the MCA Service we have had no cases of postpartum hemorrhage.

In the event that a hemorrhage or other severe problem comes up we take the mother to the nearest hospital by ambulance. If it is a breech with less urgency, or, perhaps, simply a slow labor, we try to take the mother to the most cooperative hospital even though it may be somewhat further away than the nearest one. One thing we do not do at home is deliver breech presentations. When we do go to the hospital, we always try to go where the hospital will let us come in and stay with the mother and give her support during labor even though we are not allowed to deliver babies in any of the area hospitals.

Arrangements with the hospitals for any particular woman are always made in advance. In fact, that is part of her contract and is her responsibility. The client also makes the arrangement, in advance, with the ambulance service. She posts the numbers by her phone of the ambulance service, the hospital nearest, and the hospital of her preference should it become a matter of elective admission rather than one of urgency. It is also her responsibility to find a pediatrician to see the baby at home within 24 hours. If a mother does not do these things, we will not consider her for a homebirth because the whole business of having your baby at home is that you have to be very responsible, yourself, for the care that you are getting.

One of the unique things about our service is that about half of our clients are delivered by the baby's father rather than the nurse midwife. We have taught people who have never seen a delivery how to deliver a lady over an intact perineum. It really can be done very easily. Another unique aspect we hope to add in the near future is the services of a pediatric nurse practitioner. We would like to have this as part of our service so that we can see the whole family and treat everyone.

We are absolutely delighted with the results we have gotten so far. Most of our clients, I think, are better than satisfied. We have gotten very, very positive feedback. The remainder of this presentation will be a verbatim publication of our service as we have written it up for distribution to our clients.

DESCRIPTION OF THE M.C.A. HOMEBIRTH SERVICE

1. ### General Characteristics

The homebirth service as a part of the total service provided by the Maternity Center Associates will operate under medically approved policies and directives. These have been developed jointly with the service's physician consultants, and are in accord with the philosophy of the American College of Nurse Midwives and the goals established for this service. Approved medical directives and policies are provided in Appendix A. These policies and directives will be reviewed and evaluated regularly by both the nurse midwives and the physician consultants and appropriate changes made as necessary.

Clients of the service will be given all of their primary care by nurse midwives. Consultation with, and/or referral to, the services physician consultants, or other medical specialists, will be obtained as required. Obstetrical clients routinely will be seen in the office at the frequency of one visit per month up to 28 weeks gestation; two visits per month up to 36

weeks, and then four visits per month up to term. Intrapartum
services will be provided at home, if the client meets the selection criteria, or in the hospital, in which case care will be
provided by the nurse midwife and the physician working together.
One prenatal home visit will also be included for those clients
who plan to deliver at home. Postpartum visits include visits
to the home or hospital on days one and/or two, a two-week, six-
week, six-month, and one-year visit in the office. Routine gyne-
cologic care will also be provided. Appropriate diagnostic services will be utilized as required at either the Washington
Hospital Center in the District or the Holy Cross Hospital in
Silver Spring, MD. These will include sonogram, X-ray, and laboratory services. Policies and procedures for management of the
antenatal course by the nurse midwives, which have been approved
by the medical consultants, are included in Appendix B.

Teaching on an individual basis will be included as part of the
service and clients will receive specific instruction relative
to preparations necessary for homebirth (see Appendix C). In
addition, all obstetrical clients will be encouraged to enroll
in Childbirth Education Classes offered in the Metropolitan Area.
Postpartum clients will be encouraged to take advantage of community resources for new parents.

2. Medical Direction

    Two board certified obstetricians provide the medical direction
    for the service. Their obligations include:

        (1) the delegation of responsibility for the management
             of the care of clients accepted into the service;

        (2) the review and approval of standards of care, clinical
             practice policies, and nurse midwifery orders;

        (3) the provision of consultation for clients who develop
             deviations or complications; and

        (4) the acceptance of medical responsibility for hospi-
             talization or medical referral of clients.

3. Description of the Selection and Management of Homebirth Clients

    A. Criteria for Selection of Clients

        Homebirth clients will be selected carefully according to
    specific criteria. The criteria, which are outlined below,
    have been established not only for initial acceptance but also
    for the entire prenatal period and labor. If any of the cri-
    teria is not met, the client will not be delivered at home and
    appropriate plans and/or interventions will be made. If the
    client cannot be delivered at home, one of the consulting obste-
    tricians will assume direct responsibility for the patient. In
    most instances, the physician and the nurse midwife will jointly
    manage the client under these circumstances.

Potential homebirth clients must be initially self-selected. They must expressly request a homebirth and must give evidence of sufficient commitment. Alternatives to a homebirth will be discussed with the clients, and information regarding the nature of obstetrical services in local hospitals, including "in & out" deliveries, will be provided. The risks of a homebirth will be thoroughly discussed. If the client continues to desire a home delivery, the criterion of "self-selection" will be considered to be met.

Clients must meet several nonmedical criteria in order to be accepted for a homebirth. These include:

* living within 10 miles of a hospital;

* agreeing to the transfer of self and/or the infant to a hospital if determined necessary by the attending nurse midwife or consulting physician;

* locating a pediatrician who will agree to see the newborn within 24 hours of birth;

* attending prepared childbirth classes or receiving private instructions;

* agreeing to make required preparations at home (see Appendix B).

The history, physical examination, and laboratory results of clients requesting a homebirth must be within normal limits. Normal limits is defined as no evidence of any of the following:

* hypertension
* epilepsy
* active syphilis
* active T.B.
* Rh negative with positive titers
* severe anemia
* severe psychiatric disease
* diabetes
* heart disease
* kidney disease
* multiple gestation
* pre-eclampsia
* abnormal vaginal bleeding
* unusual or abnormal presentations or lies
* previous C-section

Additionally, clients must be no younger than 15 nor older than 42 and must be no more than a gravida 5. Clients accepted for homebirth must appear emotionally mature and stable. Every primigravida will be evaluated clinically (and by X-ray pelvimetry, if necessary) to rule out CPD.

Clients for homebirth must have a normal antepartum period. This means no evidence of any of the following:

* abnormal bleeding

* pre-eclampsia

* congenital abnormalities

* inappropriate gestational size

* multiple gestation

* unusual presentation or lie

Criteria have been established for labor initiation. Labor must begin within 24 hours of rupture of membranes. The fetal head must be engaged in the primigravida. The fetus must be in a vertex position and there must be no sign of infection. Failure to meet any of these criteria requires that the client deliver in the hospital rather than at home.

B. Management of the Homebirth

As agreed when accepted as a homebirth client, the client assumes several specific responsibilities to prepare for the birth of her baby at home. These include having all necessary supplies available (see Appendix B for supplies list), selecting a pediatrician who will see the infant within 24 hours of birth, making maps to the home, and taking childbirth classes.

The nurse midwife makes a home visit approximately two weeks before the delivery date. At this time, the arrangements made by the client and the physical environment can be assessed and the expected course of the home confinement can be discussed in the surroundings where it will occur.

Once labor has begun and meets the criteria noted above, the nurse midwife will manage the labor and the delivery. She will notify the obstetrician on call at the onset of labor and will consult with him, or the pediatrician chosen by the client, as necessary. Policies and procedures for the management of the homebirth, which have been approved by the medical consultants, are included in Appendix D. Supplies and equipment which the nurse midwife will take to the home are listed in Appendix E.

Criteria have been established so that other than normal progress of the labor will require medical intervention with possible transfer to a hospital. The following situations will require such action:

* fetus in an abnormal presentation

* meconium-stained amniotic fluid

* fetal heart irregularities

* prolonged labor using criteria established by E. Friedman

* abnormal bleeding

* unengaged vertex in the primigravida

* ruptured membranes over 24 hours

* wishes of the client

In the management of the immediate postpartum period, the nurse midwife will stay with the mother and infant until vital signs are normal, the uterus is well contracted, and the baby is nursing well and shows no signs of distress. A minimum of one hour is required. If any of the following should occur, medical consultation is required with possible transfer of mother and/or baby to a hospital:

* hemorrhage

* retained products of conceptus

* laceration beyond second degree

* an infant with

  † weight less than 2,500 gm

  † respiratory difficulties

  † cardiac irregularities

  † congenital abnormalities

  † Apgar score less than 7 at 5 minutes

  † prematurity, dysmaturity, and postmaturity as determined by physical assessment

Postpartum instructions will be given to each client (see Appendix F). The nurse-midwife will make postpartum visits to the family on day 1 and/or 2 to evaluate the condition of mother and baby. The infant will be seen by the family's pediatrician within 24 hours of birth. The mother will be seen in the office by the nurse midwife at 2 and 6 weeks postpartum. The nurse midwife will complete and sign the birth certificate.

C. Description of Backup Resources

In the event that any aspect of the homebirth does not meet the criteria established as normal or, if in the nurse midwife's judgement assistance is required, the nurse-midwife will have appropriate resources available. In every homebirth instance, the obstetrician on call will be notified of the onset of labor and will be available for telephone and/or on-site consultation. A pediatrician, chosen by the client, will also be available for consultation if a problem develop with the infant.

If mother or baby requires hospitalization, the obstetrician or pediatrician will admit the client to the hospital. The physicians who are medical consultants to the service have hospital privileges at the following hospitals:

* Georgetown University Hospital

* Washington Hospital Center

* Sibley Hospital

* Fairfax Hospital

* Alexandria Hospital

If the situation requiring hospitalization is of an emergency nature and does not allow time for transfer to one of the above hospitals, the client will be transported to the nearest hospital. Since the above-mentioned hospitals will be easily accessible for most clients accepted for homebirth, this situation is not likely to occur. In an emergency, the clients will be transported by rescue squad, otherwise by private ambulance or car. The nurse midwife will accompany the client to the hospital.

AΩAΩAΩAΩAΩAΩAΩAΩAΩAΩAΩAΩAΩAΩAΩAΩAΩAΩAΩAΩAΩAΩAΩAΩAΩAΩAΩAΩAΩAΩAΩAΩAΩAΩAΩAΩ

APPENDIX A

MEDICATION DIRECTIVES

(OR STANDING ORDERS)

Medications prescribed by the physician and approved for issue by the nurse midwife are as follows:

Antepartum

1. Bendectin tabs 2@ h.s. and tab 1 or 2 in A.M.

2. Ferrous fumarate tab 1 TID

3. Vitron C. tabs 2 daily

4. Folic acid 1 mg daily

5. Multivitamins

6. Vaginal infection therapy

   1. Floraquin Vag Tabs
   2. Tri-mo-san
   3. Nystatin
   4. Sporostacin
   5. Monistat IX/day
   6. Vanobid
   7. Sultrin
   8. Aci-jel
   9. AVC with Dinestrol

APPENDIX A CONT'D
(STANDING ORDERS)

7. Douches

   1. Ivory Liquid
   2. Vinegar
   3. Betadine
   4. Over-the-Counter

8. Laxatives

   1. Over-the-Counter
   2. Lomotil

9. Antacids - Over-the Counter

10. Antibiotics (check for allergies)

    1. Gantrisin or AZO - Gantrisin 500 mg tabs 2 qid
    2. Ampicillin 500 mg q 4 hrs. x 10 days

11. Decongestants

    1. Over-the-Counter
    2. Actifed, Naldecon, Triaminic 1 tab TID

12. Cough Medicine

    1. Robitussin DM - Over-the-Counter
    2. Phenergan VC Expec with Codeine 1 tsp of 4 to 6 hrs.

Intrapartum

1. Local infiltration with Xylocaine 1% up to 30 cc.

2. Repair episiotomy with chromic $\frac{..}{oo}$

3. Prep and enema (Fleets) PRN

Postpartum

1. Pitocin 10u to 20u IM or IV after delivery or after placenta as indicated

2. IV fluids for hydration

   1. 5% D/W
   2. 5% D/.45 NaCl

3. IV fluids of choice with no more than 40u of Pitocin as indicated for excessive bleeding postpartum with consultation

4. Ergotrate gr 1/320 IM x 1 for uterine atony in absence of hypertension

5. Ergotrate p.o. 0.02 mg x 6 doses

6. Empirin compd #3 tabs 1 q 3-4 hrs PRN for pain

7. Darvoset N tabs 2 q 4 hrs PRN for pain

8. Equanil 400 mg for sleep

9. Iron and vitamins: see antepartum orders

APPENDIX A CONT'D
(STANDING ORDERS)

10. Antibiotics: see antepartum orders

11. Laxatives: see antepartum orders

12. Decongestants and cough medicines: see antepartum orders

13. Vaginal infection therapy: see antepartum orders

14. Family Planning

    1. Oral contraceptives
    2. IUD: CU-7, Lippes Loop, Saf-T-Coil
    3. Diaphragm
    4. Foam and condoms
    5. Rhythm - Basal Temp.

Laboratory examinations may be requested as appropriate:

1. T and Cx

2. Type, Rh, Antibody screen

3. Repeat antibody studies

4. CBC and/or H and H (< 10 requires consultation)

5. VDRL

6. Cultures and sensitivities

7. Urinalysis

8. Rhogam studies

9. Pap smears

10. Rubella titers

11. Sonogram

12. Pelvimetry

For More Information
On This Homebirth Service
Write:

MATERNITY CENTER ASSOCIATES, LTD.
5415 Cedar Lane, Suite 107-B
Bethesda, Maryland 20014

APPENDIX B

ANTEPARTUM POLICIES AND DIRECTIVES

I. Nurse Midwives will provide care for:

A. CNM Service clients

B. Non-CNM Service clients (clients who are referred for CNM care by a physician)

II. Antepartum Management:

A. Initial Screening History and Physical Examination

B. Routine antepartum visits every 4 weeks until the 28th week of gestation; every 2 weeks until the 36th week; every week thereafter

C. Procedures:

1. Complete history at first visit

2. Complete physical examination at first visit, including:

   a. EENT screening
   b. heart and lungs
   c. abdominal palpation (including liver and spleen)
   d. pelvic examination (including clinical pelvimetry)
   e. laboratory procedures:

      1. Type, Rh, antibody screen
      2. VDRL
      3. CBC
      4. Rubella titer
      5. Routine urinalysis
      6. Pap Smear
      7. G.C. culture

3. Pelvic examination as necessary or as requested by client throughout antepartum course

4. B/P, weight, urinalysis (for glucose and protein), and abdominal examination (Leopold's maneuvers) at every antepartum visit

D. Directives:

1. The nurse midwife must consult with the physician regarding any finding which appears abnormal on the history or physical examination.

2. The nurse midwife may treat vaginal infections diagnosed by wet smear or culture with the appropriate medication without consultation.

3. The nurse midwife may use medications as listed under "Medication Directives" (Appendix A) as deemed necessary.

APPENDIX B CONT'D
(ANTEPARTUM POLICIES)

4. The physician must be consulted in cases of:
    a. Urinary tract infections
    b. Positive gonorrhea cultures
    c. Positive VDRL titers
    d. Hemoglobin of less than 10.0 (Hemoglobin of less than 10.0 must be treated with Ferrous Fumarate or Vitron C as indicated)
    e. Rising antibody titers
        1. Rh
        2. Rubella

APPENDIX C

PRENATAL INSTRUCTIONS

SUPPLIES NEEDED FOR MOTHER AND DELIVERY

* A stiff bed is best, use plywood under mattress if necessary
* Plastic mattress cover or inexpensive shower curtain to protect mattress
* Optional: plastic pillow cases to protect pillows
* Small pile of newspapers
* Plastic-lined trash receptacle
* Glad or Giant brand bags (plastic, leak-proof, 18 qt size)
* Bowl with a rounded bottom for the placenta
* Roll of paper towels
* 2 dozen 4" x 4" gauze pads
* 1 bottle Zephiran Chloride 1:750
* Fleets enema
* Chux bed pads (Sears or Wards under pads are less expensive, but must be ordered from catalog. It takes about 10-14 days)
* 4 oz. ear syringe
* Scissors
* White shoestrings
* Two maps useful to find place at night
* A place for nurse midwife to sit and/or lie down for rest
* Clean towels and washcloths
* Sanitary belt
* Hospital-size sanitary napkins
* Clean gown or pajamas

SUPPLIES NEEDED FOR THE INFANT

* One or two old receiving blankets
* Hair brush
* Diapers, pins, shirt and gown or kimono to dress the baby
* Clean blankets
* Rectal thermometer
* Cotton balls
* Alcohol
* Scales (bathroom scales may be used)
* Tape measure (optional)
* Clean towels and washcloths
* Bed for baby

APPENDIX C CONT'D
(PRENATAL INSTRUCTIONS)

GENERAL INSTRUCTIONS

* Check with the midwife a few weeks prior to your delivery date and she will give you instructions regarding the prenatal home visit and when she is to be notified.

* It is wise to preregister and tour the hospital you would use as an alternative to homebirth. Also, pack a bag in the event that hospitalization is necessary.

* Select a pediatrician who will agree to see your baby within the first 24 hours after delivery either at your home or in his office. Give the pediatrician's name and telephone number to the nurse midwife two weeks prior to the delivery date.

* Have all supplies ready three weeks before delivery date.

* Take classes in Preparation for Childbirth.

* Make up delivery bed in the following manner:

  A. Cover for mattress, if desired
  B. Clean fitted sheet
  C. Plastic mattress cover or shower curtain
  D. Clean fitted sheet

* After delivery, the top fitted sheet and plastic mattress cover are removed and a clean fitted sheet is then readily available on the bed.

TELEPHONE NUMBERS

* Janet Epstein   299-8377 or 8378

* Marion McCartney   966-6856

* Office & Answering Service 530-9199

* It is wise to call the Office/Answering Service first. They will tell you who is on call and where she may be reached.

BIRTH CERTIFICATE

* The nurse midwife will complete and sign your baby's birth certificate.

APPENDIX D

LABOR AND DELIVERY POLICIES AND DIRECTIVES

I. Nurse Midwives will provide care for:

   A. CNM Service clients

   B. Non-CNM Service clients (clients who are referred for CNM care by a physician)

II. Labor Management - First Stage. Support and management will include the following:

   A. Labor Policies

      1. May evaluate labor of the client by performing vaginal examinations.
      2. May execute physical exam, including heart and lung evaluation.
      3. Pelvic evaluation by the CNM as indicated.
      4. Will consult physician whenever necessary during labor.
      5. Will request medical management for any medical or obstetrical complication.
      6. Request admission to hospital of the client to the delivery suite when indicated. Must consult with physician.

   B. Vital Signs

      1. Temperature, Pulse, Respirations as necessary.
      2. BP as indicated
      3. FHT q 30 min. routinely, or more frequently during second stage.

   C. Evaluation of Progress

      1. Abdominal palpation.
      2. Evaluation of contractions for intensity, duration, and frequency.
      3. Vaginal and/or rectal examinations.
      4. Behavioral changes and/or physical changes.

   D. Procedures

      1. Routine laboratory procedures done antenatally:

         a. Type, Rh
         b. CBC
         c. VDRL
         d. Urine tested for protein and glucose
         e. Nitrazine test if indicated

      2. Ambulation at discretion of nurse midwife.
      3. Enema: may be given at discretion of nurse midwife after evaluating condition of cervix, station of presenting part, and progress of labor and preference of client.
      4. Intravenous infusion, if necessary.
      5. Amniotomy if indicated. Criteria:
         a. Active labor
         b. Vertex presenting with head engaged
         c. 3-4 cm dilated

APPENDIX D CONT'D
(LABOR POLICIES)

E. Notification of physician for:

    1. Any bleeding other than show
    2. Fetal distress
    3. Maternal distress
    4. Prolonged stages of labor
    5. Elevation of temperature of blood pressure
    6. Prolonged ROM

III. Delivery Management

    A. Vital Signs

        1. FHT q 5 minutes or as indicated

    B. Evaluation of progress - physician to be notified of
        prolonged second stage.

    C. Prolonged third stage

        1. Placenta retained for more than thirty minutes without
            bleeding.

    D. Procedures

        1. Amniotomy
        2. Local infiltration of perineum
        3. Episiotomy and repair
        4. Cervical inspection
        5. Manual removal of placenta when necessary
        6. Manual exploration of uterus, when necessary

    E. Medications (See Medication Directives, Appendix A)

        1. Xylocaine Hydrochloride 1% for local infiltration
        2. Oxytocin
            a. 10u. -20 u IM or IV after birth of baby and/or
                placenta, as indicated, or
            b. 10u. -40 u in IV bottle after delivery of placenta,
                as indicated.
        3. Methergine 0.2 mg IM or after delivery of placenta as
            indicated for PPH, if no evidence of hypertension.
        4. Ergotrate 1/320 IM in absence of hypertension.

IV. Newborn Management

    A. Routine Procedures
        1. Suction
        2. Care of cord
        3. Apgar Score
        4. AgNO$_3$
        5. Aquamephyton upon order of pediatrician

    B. Resuscitative measure as indicated
        1. Mouth-to-mouth using infant airway
        2. Insufflation with Ambubag

APPENDIX D CONT'D
(LABOR POLICIES)

V. <u>Immediate Postpartum</u>

    A. All of the postpartum medication directives hold for the client in the immediate postpartum period. Also included are routine 2-week and 6-week checkups and family planning services.

    B. Cord blood will be collected from all Rh negative mothers and sent to the laboratory for the appropriate studies. (Rhogam will be administered by the laboratory when necessary.)

APPENDIX E

MIDWIVES' SUPPLIES & MEDICATIONS

1. Episiotomy Set:

    a. 1 Kelly Clamp;
    b. 1 Bandage Scissor (Large);
    c. Medium Needle Holder;
    d. Sterile 4" x 4" gauze dressings.

2. BP Cuff and Stethoscope

3. Fetoscope

4. Ambubag (infant size)

5. Amnihooks

6. Ear Syringe (4 oz.)

7. Zephiran Chloride 1:750

8. Suture 00 Chromic (#983 or #811)

9. Medications:

    a. 100cc 5% D/W or 100cc 5% D/.45 NaCl
    b. Pitocin 10U/1cc
    c. Methergine Ampules
    d. Ergotrate Ampules
    e. Silver Nitrate and Aquamephyton

10. Needles, Syringes, Alcohol, Sponges

11. Uristix

12. Birth Certificate forms

13. Labor and Delivery records

14. Postpartum Instructions

15. Two red top and 1 blue top blood tubes (for cord blood on Rh negative mothers)

APPENDIX F

POSTPARTUM INSTRUCTIONS

1. Call the office (530-9199) and make an appointment to see the nurse midwife 2 weeks and 6 weeks from delivery date.

2. No shopping or anything tiring for about 2 weeks.

3. Exercises (may begin one day after delivery)
   a. KEGEL - start immediately by contracting muscles of the pelvic floor.
   b. Situps - Start with one in the morning and one in the afternoon.
   c. Leg lifts - Work up to 10 a day.

4. Call the pediatrician and make an appointment for the baby to be seen within the first 24 hours after delivery.

5. Feel free to call us if you have any problems that you wish to discuss.

6. Nurse the baby frequently. Do not bathe until the cord has dried up or the circumcision is healed. (Make an appointment with Dr. Brew or Dr. DeVocht if you want your baby circumsized.) The cord does not require any special care.

AS LONG AS THE SITUATION REMAINS NORMAL, OUR CLIENTS CAN DO AND SUGGEST ALMOST ANYTHING. ALTHOUGH THESE APPENDICES LIST NUMEROUS MEDICAL DIRECTIVES OF WHICH WE MAY HAVE NEED IF INDICATED, THESE ARE OPENLY DISCUSSED AND PRESENTED TO THE CLIENT ANTEPARTUM AND ARE NEVER CALLED UPON WITHOUT THE UNDERSTANDING, CONSENT, AND CONSIDERATION OF THE PERSONAL PREFERENCES OF THE CLIENT. WE CONSIDER OURSELVES AS HIRED EXPERTS--ONLY THERE TO HELP AND TO MONITOR THINGS SO THAT EVERYTHING GOES WELL.

CLIENT INFORMATION SHEET

SILVER NITRATE

Q. Why must silver nitrate be used in the baby's eyes after birth?

A. 1% solution of silver nitrate is the recommended prophylactic treatment for prevention of gonorrheal ophthalmia (blindness due to gonorrheal infection contracted from the mother's birth canal) in newborns. In Maryland, Virginia and the District of Columbia, it is the law and a nurse midwife can lose her license for failure to treat the newborn.

Q. Why not test the mother for gonorrhea and only treat those babies who need it?

A. Two reasons:

1. Although testing is available, results are unreliable. Both the method of obtaining the cultures and failure to incubate immediately (lack of facilities) result in many false negatives (mother has gonorrhea but it does not show up on the culture.)

2. Gonorrhea can be contracted at any time by the pregnant woman or her partner before delivery. The nurse midwife cannot be responsible for deciding who may or may not have been exposed to gonorrhea. (Think about that for a moment, please.)

Q. Why not use penicillin argerol or tetracycline which appear to be less irritating to the baby's eyes?

A. The American Academy of Pediatrics' most recent statement on this is in support of silver nitrate (it is supposed to be the most effective). They believe that the side effects are less of a disadvantage than missing a case of gonorrheal ophthalmia by a less potent drug. The laws here specify silver nitrate; no substitute is acceptable.

Q. What about the damage to the infant's eyes?

A. A chemical conjunctivitis (redness, swelling and/or discharge) can develop after using silver nitrate. These symptoms are temporary; permanent damage does not result.

Q. Does using silver nitrate interfere with bonding between the mother and infant right after birth?

A. We feel it does and in our practice we wait one hour after birth before using it. We find that the babies do not cry if they have first had a chance to look around and to nurse before we treat their eyes.

FORMS AND FORMATS

The foregoing pages have presented the details of our homebirth service including the printed materials we distribute to our clients discussing the possible medical interventions, responsibilities of the parents, delineation of the various tasks of the birth to be handled by the midwives and by themselves, as well as instructions for postpartum, the rationale of using silver nitrate, etc. In conclusion we present here some of the standard forms we use to keep adequate records on the births of our clients.

The prenatal record is tabulated on two standard forms which shall not be shown here. They are:

1. The Prenatal Record Form developed jointly by the Committee on Maternal and Child Care of the American Medical Association and the American College of Obstetricians and Gynecologists.

2. The Prenatal Hospital Form, #9801-88G: 170-500M (OP-65), available from the American Medical Association.

The format and appearence of our Standing Order Prescription Form is reproduced below (slightly reduced from actual size):

MATERNITY CENTER ASSOCIATES, LTD.
5411 CEDAR LANE
SUITE 204-A
BETHESDA, MARYLAND 20014
(301) 530-9199

James D. Brew, Jr., M.D.   Janet L. Epstein, R.N., C.N.M.
L. J. DeVocht, M.D.   Marion McCartney, R.N., C.N.M.

Name _____ Date _____

Address _____

℞

Label as to Contents

Refill .... Times

Within .... Months

Reproduced below is a facsimile of our Labor and Delivery Form slightly reduced (actual size is the standard, 8 1/2 x 11 inches).

LABOR AND DELIVERY RECORD

CENTIMETERS (O) — STATION (X)

HOURS: 0 1 2 3 4 5 6 7 8 9 10 11 12 13 14

Name: Date: Age:

Address: Telephone: EDC

G   P   AB   Blood Type:

Membranes Ruptured (Spont. or Artif.)   Problems During Pregnancy:
at:

Amniotic Fluid:
Stage   I from   to   =   Hrs
Stage II from   to   =   Min/Hrs
Stage III from   to   =   Min

                Total time
                in Labor

Delivery Information   Newborn Information

Time: Sex: Weight:

Position: Apgar 1 min.   5 min.

Cord around neck: Gross abnormalities

Perineum: Eyes treated:
                                         Aquamephyton 1 mg: Yes____   No____
Placenta:
Method   Pediatrician:
Mechanism

Estimated Blood Loss

Oxytoxic

Additional Comments:

Fourth Stage: Labor and Delivery Managed by:

                                         Maternity Center Associates, Ltd.

Our Postpartum Form is reproduced below (slightly reduced), actual size being 8 1/2 x 5 1/2 inches.

POSTPARTUM

Physical:

Weeks:

Wt. and B/P:

Bleeding:

Breasts and Nipples:

Abdomen:

Pelvic:

    Muscle Tone   Fundus

    Vulva:

    Vagina:

    Perineum:

    Cervix:

    Uterus:

    Adnexa:

    Recto-Vaginal:

Impression:

Rx:

Emotional:

Sleep:

Problems:

Infant Feeding:

Birth Control Plan: None

Pill   IUD   Diaphragm

Foam   Condom   Rhythm

Sterilization - Type

Signed: Date:

THE LAY MIDWIFE

Nancy Mills, LM*

In many countries in the world, midwifery plays a very, very major role in the health care of women. And in less industrialized countries, midwifery plays more than just the role of attending birth. It plays the part of being a community helper, a community assistant, a person who really relates to families and gets out there and does almost a social service kind of thing with the community. In these cultures, a midwife is usually very respected by the communities in which she works.

In the United States, the midwife is beginning to be accepted back, but for the most part, she is the nurse midwife--not the midwife we used to know. There is obviously a great need and the nurse midwife, I believe, is filling a role that greatly needs to be filled and has come back on the scene not a minute too soon. But the problem I see with the nurse midwife is that she is not meeting the needs in a world community. In Sonoma County, where I live in California, I am 75 miles north of San Francisco and in the communities north of me, all the way, probably to Canada, there aren't any nurse midwives. But there is an ever increasing number of lay midwives.

The lay midwife is not something that has just gotten started in this country. I began 6 years ago in Sonoma County. At the time, I was the only midwife I knew around there attending births. I could not find nor get in touch with anybody who was a lay midwife--even in San Francisco.

I read a paper by Florence Lee and Jay Glaser written about two years ago where they had collected some interesting information on the practice of midwifery in Texas and Appalachia. The lay midwives there have been practicing for about 35 years in the group they studied. The age range of the midwives was 56-65 years old. The educational level of these midwives was high school, although not all had graduated from high school. All the midwives were literate and filled out birth records. The length of time of residence in the areas where they lived for these midwives was an average of about 16 years. None of them had formal training, although many of them said that they had trained with physicians.

* NANCY MILLS is a Lay Midwife with some 6 years' experience and has attended over 350 homebirths and over 100 hospital births; she has 3 children, the first two born in hospitals and the last at home; she is founder and former President of the Northern California Midwives Association; she is a consultant to the State of California, Department of Maternal & Child Health as well as an advisor to several others engaged in research in maternity and infant care; she has been featured in several books and at least one TV Documentary by NBC TV; she is currently a Public Health Assistant, Sonoma County Public Health Department, Santa Rosa, California.

The article by Lee and Glaser went on to point out how the midwives talked about their limitations. The majority of them said that
they would like to attend some kind of training course. All of the
midwives in the study (I think there were about 20 interviewed)
stated the reasons that they attended births and they were all the
same reasons why I attend births. It's kind of interesting. Comments
were made like: "I just prefer a midwife and a home delivery."
"There was no doctor available." "I didn't like the hospital." "I
didn't want to leave my children and family." "I prefer to have a
woman with me." "I can't afford a hospital." Osgood, who wrote an
article on granny midwives in Appalachia said that in communities
where nurses, nurse midwives, and doctors were available, the lay
midwife was usually chosen *over* the professionals because mothers
felt they received better care from lay midwives in their homes.

In Madero County, California, ten years ago, the State supported a project that introduced midwives into that community. It was a
very rural, low income community and lacked availability of any prenatal care. After one year, the infant mortality was reduced from
23.9 per 1000 live births to 10.3. Prematurity dropped from 11% of
all births to 6.4%. These midwives obviously proved a great need
for health care in that particular community. The project was
dropped, at the recommendation of the Health Department and the
obstetricians of the State. Within six months, the very high percentage of problems increased back to its normal of its unusually
high rate that existed before the program was adopted.

I mentioned that I started midwifery about 6 years ago in
Sonoma County. I had never thought about being a midwife. I had had
two children at the time. They are now ages 12 and 13. I had an
interesting experience with my first birth because I was under age
and the doctor thought that he could not legally give me an anesthetic. So I went to the hospital in labor and he came into my room and
said," Well, I am not going to give you any pain medication, but
you are really young and you're going to have an easy time and don't
worry about it." And I said, "Okay." Later I went into the delivery
room and had a remarkably easy time and just went away with a very
beautiful experience, not knowing much of anything at the time. Well,
in the next few years I had the opportunity to talk to quite a few
friends and my sister, who had a baby, and heard them all tell me
stories about how they didn't feel a thing. In my own personal birth
experience, I had had such a wonderful time giving birth. It felt so
great that I was really upset and concerned about women not feeling
their birth. I wasn't familiar with Marshall Klaus at the time and I
wasn't familiar with all the studies that are out now talking about
how important it is that we do feel and do experience our birth. But
something told me that this was an important thing.

The way I became involved in midwifery some years after I had
my first two children was very accidental. I was actually walking
down the road one afternoon along the river and stopped in to see a
friend. This friend happened to be in labor. I didn't know she
was in labor, but her husband was very frantic and said, "Would you
please run down to the store and phone the doctor because we need

some advice." So I did and the doctor told me, "Bring her into the hospital." I went back and said, "You have to go into the hospital," and she said, "No, I won't go. I had my last baby there and it was horrible and I'm going to stay home." Well, not knowing a thing about it, I was a little concerned because I knew the doctor. He was my family doctor and seemed like a reasonable person to me. I was a little worried but I stuck around and helped her husband who was having a pretty hard time of it and we delivered the baby. It was really a beautiful experience for me. I kind of came away from it saying, "Well, you know, that's the kind of experience I had and this is the first I know about where the woman had a similar experience to myself."

Well, about two weeks later a friend of this lady's called, who I didn't know, and said, "Gee, Linda told me about how great a help you were at her birth and how you came back and helped her for the next few days and I'm going to have my baby at home. Do you think you could come down and help me out since you are the only one in the neighborhood who has seen a baby born?" So I did. And everything went okay. And when it comes right down to it, I've done about 400 since then and all have gone pretty much the same way.

IN COMMUNITIES WHERE NURSES, NURSE MIDWIVES, AND DOCTORS ARE AVAILABLE, THE LAY MIDWIFE IS OFTEN CHOSEN OVER THE PROFESSIONAL BECAUSE MOTHERS FEEL THEY RECEIVE BETTER CARE.

My experiences were positive and I think that for a midwife, that is really important initially. The first 10 or 12 births that I attended, I had no problems. There were no complications that required me to take a woman to the hospital. I am sure that was a great benefit to me and I am thankful that we didn't come up with any major problems that frightened me. Because of this I was able to begin from the start to see birth as a normal, natural physiological event in the home. Most of the complications I saw were when I took a woman into the hospital.

In the hospital, not only were the women often mistreated and misdiagnosed but humiliated to the point that I found myself in tears many a time in an emergency room holding a woman's hand who was just literally being messed over by some doctor who was really angry that she had had her baby at home or that she was in labor and had attempted to have her baby at home. I saw very soon that most of the complications and interference were in the hospital. At home we didn't have too many problems.

Initially, I had no support. I had no physician backup. There was just nothing there for me to do. I sometimes felt I almost had to make the choice to stay home even with the problem in order to avoid a more serious problem if we went to the hospital.

IN A RURAL, LOW INCOME COUNTY IN CALIFORNIA, THE STATE ONCE SUPPORTED A PROGRAM OF MIDWIVES WHICH, AFTER ONE YEAR, RESULTED IN REDUCING THE RATES OF INFANT MORTALITY AND PREMATURITY BY APPROXIMATELY 50%. THE PROJECT WAS LATER DROPPED UPON THE RECOMMENDATIONS OF THE HEALTH DEPARTMENT AND THE OBSTETRICIANS OF THE STATE AND THE MORTALITY AND PREMATURITY RATES SOON RETURNED TO THEIR FORMER HIGH VALUES.

There was quite a bit of anger and resentment in the community initially. In the second to third year that I was working as a midwife, I was attending up to 15 births a month. The local obstetricians got pretty uptight about it. They called upon the State Board of Medical Examiners who paid me a visit and presented me with a Cease and Desist Order that would lead to prosecution if I didn't follow it. So I just sort of smiled at the man and he went away.

I continued attending some births but kind of slowed down for a while and put a lot of energy into working as a patient advocate. Largely, I see the role of the midwife as a patient advocate, as a protector of women and a protector of babies. I started trying to get into the hospital more and talk to people more. I got involved in writing a grant in 1971. I met a fine nurse who was interested in doing her Masters Thesis on homebirth. She came out and dug me up out in the woods somewhere and we sat down and had a long talk about it. She then started attending home visits with me--not births, just visits. We started collecting some sociodemographic information on the people and asking them questions about why they were having their babies at home. This led to the writing of a grant which was funded by the State of California, Department of Maternal and Child Health. The name of the grant became known as the "Maternity Outreach Project." For one year we collected statistics and did a survey of the results which went back to the State. We found that in the particular area that I was in the incidence of homebirths was much higher than any of the other counties in the Bay Area at the time. As we worked with this study we managed to find some other lay midwives around and found that the incidence of homebirth was also increasing in other counties in the Bay Area.

The second year of the grant we reported to the State that there was an increasing incidence of homebirth and a very high percentage of these women had no prenatal care at all. In the area we were in, it could be up to two hours' drive to Santa Rosa--the town with the nearest available obstetrical care or residency program. So women were just not coming in. Also that second year, we established a clinic out in the Russian River area. With the little bit of money that they gave us, we continued to study and we set up a clinic in an old house and a midwife (who wasn't a nurse) who was actually a certified midwife from Ireland, but not registered in California because, at the time, midwifery wasn't legal.

The Irish midwife and I worked together for about a year. She taught me a lot about prenatal care. This was about 4 years ago. We did all our own prenatal care and couldn't find a doctor to come and work out in our clinic. Finally, one nice GP said, "Well, I don't deliver babies at home and I have no connection with a hospital so I can't even help you there, but I'll come out to the clinic and be there to sign your charts and make your clinic legal that way." So he came on out and didn't know much about prenatal care but signed our charts.

In that first year, we managed to have a pretty good outcome in our births at home. We never had a fetal death or a maternal death and our outcomes were looking good. The State Department of Health became very interested in us because they were also seeing an extremely high incidence of homebirth all over the State of California. Since we were the only homebirth research project that had been funded, they decided to kind of step up our project and give us some more money in order to ask us for a lot more information. So we have been funded every year and are continuing to gather the sociodemographic information on people and really expanding our project. We have been also working with Lewis Mehl some too as well as with Marshall Klaus on the mother-infant bonding research.

Through the years one of the things that we have managed to accomplish, which I am very pleased about, is that we have a family practice residency program in Santa Rosa. There are 28 residents that come up from U.C. in San Francisco or from other universities, actually from all over, and come into Santa Rosa where they spend 3 years in family practice. In the last couple of years, quite a few of them have expressed a great interest towards our program. So we've managed to get them into our clinics on a fulltime basis in the last year. We now have four family practice residents who rotate through the clinic, seeing patients every other month.

WHEN I HAD TO TAKE A WOMAN TO THE HOSPITAL, NOT ONLY WAS SHE OFTEN MISTREATED AND MISDIAGNOSED, BUT SHE WAS OFTEN HUMILIATED TO THE POINT THAT I FOUND MYSELF IN TEARS MANY A TIME IN AN EMERGENCY ROOM HOLDING A WOMAN'S HAND WHO WAS JUST LITERALLY BEING MESSED OVER BY SOME DOCTOR WHO WAS REALLY ANGRY THAT SHE HAD HAD HER BABY AT HOME OR THAT SHE WAS IN LABOR AND HAD ATTEMPTED TO HAVE HER BABY AT HOME.

The care and routine in the clinic includes pretty much the same things presented elsewhere in this book for homebirth mothers: regular monthly visits up to 34 weeks, and then every two weeks, and then every week in the last month. We do nutrition histories when the woman comes in and nutrition counseling on the very first visit. On the second visit, we do a complete physical examination, and because the clinic has been operating for four years now, women are coming in during the first and second months of pregnancy. We do pregnancy testing too. We also have a family planning clinic and a well-baby clinic. We have a check-off list to remind us of all the things we need to discuss with the patient.

50% of the women that come in to us request a homebirth. We do not propose homebirth. We do not encourage homebirth. But we do have an increasing high incidence of homebirth. Our philosophy is that a woman has a right to a choice of where she gives birth and we do not make this decision or make the suggestion to her. Many of the doctors in Sonoma County say, "If we could get rid of Nancy Mills, we wouldn't have this problem." Well, I really disagree. They can get rid of me, but they will then just have to get out there and do it themselves.

INITIALLY, WHEN I HAD NO PHYSICIAN SUPPORT, I SOMETIMES FELT THAT I HAD TO MAKE THE CHOICE OF STAYING HOME WITH A PROBLEM IN ORDER TO AVOID A MORE SERIOUS PROBLEM IF WE WENT IN TO AN UNFRIENDLY HOSPITAL.

We do pretty much a complete lab work on all of our patients. We do a GC culture, we do Pap smears, we do everything that a regular OB practice does, but we do a few more things. We go to the home for a visit. I think one of the most critical parts of the care we have to offer is our home visiting aspects. We do *several* home visits before the birth to get to know the families. And we do this whether they are planning their baby in the hospital or in the home so that when labor comes, we are ready to go to the hospital and "labor coach" or to the home. We want to feel like we know the family, we want to know who is there. We discuss preparation for homebirth. We discuss having help there with the children and the kind of backup they are going to have. We talk to them about whether they feel confident in their doctor, whether they will go to the hospital if we recommend that they go. And this is something I feel very strongly about: I have had patients whom I have recommended to go into the hospital during the course of labor who have refused to go. It can become a difficult situation at times. One thing we do discuss is the risks and the responsibilities of homebirth--and I stress *responsibility*. There are some people who are irresponsible.

THE LOCAL OBSTETRICIANS GOT PRETTY UPTIGHT AND CALLED THE STATE BOARD OF MEDICAL EXAMINERS WHO PAID ME A VISIT AND PRESENTED ME WITH A CEASE AND DESIST ORDER THAT WOULD LEAD TO PROSECUTION IF I DIDN'T FOLLOW IT. SO I JUST SORT OF SMILED AT THE MAN AND HE WENT AWAY AND I CONTINUED ATTENDING BIRTHS.

I do not routinely use silver nitrate. In some cases I leave it up to my own perceptions and my own feelings, intuition about that family and whether or not I feel comfortable about questioning them about it. But I do advise everyone as to the use and need for silver nitrate. We did have one case about 4 years ago, a baby who did get infected and was hospitalized. An experience like that can be pretty shattering and I really found myself, at that point, using silver nitrate more. But I try very hard to respect the wishes of families and pretty much be as flexible as I can.

We do postpartum care. We do family planning. We discourage
the use of IUD's because they're hazardous to your health. We discourage the use of oral contraceptives for the same reasons. And
we have a lot of happy women using diaphragms. I'd also like to be
able to get into a place where we could start working with women
when they are   preteenagers and get them to learn a little more
about the responsibility they need to take for their bodies so that
when the time comes, they are ready to accept the responsibility
that goes along with using a diaphragm rather than using something
that is bad for you.

We do screen our patients. Our criteria are pretty much the
same as are discussed elsewhere in this book. We will not attend a
high risk mother at home. Part of the reason the statistics on homebirth do look so good is because the problems go to the hospitals.
One of the doctors in Marin County got kicked off the staff of the
local hospital because his statistics looked bad. But the only
babies he delivered in the hospital were problems. He had to go in
and explain that all of his normal births, which were about 96%,
occurred at home.

MANY OF THE DOCTORS IN SONOMA COUNTY SAY, "IF WE COULD GET
RID OF NANCY MILLS, WE WOULDN'T HAVE THE HOMEBIRTH PROBLEM."
WELL, THEY CAN GET RID OF ME, BUT THEN THEY WILL JUST HAVE TO GET
OUT THERE AND DO IT THEMSELVES.

In recent years I have been reading everything I could on
nurse midwifery and lay midwifery. Recently, I read an article
called, "Homebirth--Myth and Message" by a certified nurse midwife.
The principle objection raised in this article by health professionals against homebirth was not that it was *unsafe*, but that it
was *uneconomical* from the perspective of the professional. Some of
the reasons stated were that time was lost in travel and that only
one individual at a time could be cared for in the home while several patients could be cared for simultaneously in the hospital.
Also stated was that too much professional time would be spent
"inactive" and on call in the home. My response to hearing and
reading this was that our concern for money seems to be greater
than our concern for quality of care.

Personally, I have never felt idle at home. I see myself as
going in and being a helper, being an attendant. Sometimes it means
that I sit near the room. Sometimes I play with the kids or I do
some cooking. Sometimes I sit with the woman. Sometimes I help
a husband assist the woman. Some families need more help than
others but it's easy to go in and see how you can fit in and see
where you are needed and how you can fill that role.

I now have three children of my own. The two oldest are 12
and 13 and I have a little boy who's five who I delivered at home
myself with the help of my husband and my other two children. In
that experience, I sat up and pretty much attended my own birth.
My husband helped me and it was kind of funny. I handed him the

baby and he didn't quite know what to do. My friend, who was there,
said, "Well, cut the cord." And he cut the cord. I guess I wasn't
paying attention. I think I was talking to my daughter about why I
was crying, trying to explain to her that it was because I was happy
and not that I was sad. The baby got wrapped in a blanket and put
into my arms and as I peeled the blanket off, as every woman does
when she first gets her baby in her arms, the cord fell out and it
was about 15 inches long! I guess that was better than cutting it
too short.

        My own experience at home with women, and this is something
I have more or less tested out, especially over the last year, is
that whenever I am there labor progresses and when I leave, it often
stops. Whenever I have gone to a home and a woman is only a centi-
meter or two dilated and I sat down for a few minutes and maybe
talked with her explaining about where she was at in her labor and
then deciding that I had something more important to do and left,
telling her that I would return later, I usually came back and
found her in about the same place. Because of this, I had to
question what my role really was and what my need at that home
really was. I have come to realize that if I didn't leave, or when
I did return after having left, labor would usually pick up and
proceed at a fairly good rate. So in staying there, I think that
it makes labor at home shorter. In fact, I think that there has
been a study now that shows that homebirths are shorter. I know
that in my own statistics on homebirths, the labors I have attended
have very definitely been shorter. So the midwife is playing a
very important role. It is important for that woman to be able to
look at you, to know you are there, to hold your hand, to be reas-
sured. I know it helps when I can say to a woman, "I know how you
feel. I know it's harder than you thought it was going to be, but
you can do it." It is a very important thing that women should not
be left alone in labor--either in a hospital or at home.

WE DISCOURAGE THE USE OF IUD'S AND ORAL CONTRACEPTIVES
BECAUSE THEY ARE HAZARDOUS TO YOUR HEALTH,   WE   HAVE
A LOT OF HAPPY WOMEN USING DIAPHRAGMS.

        Well, birth is increasing regardless of what anybody does
about it and the costs are increasing greatly too. One of the problems with nurse midwifery is that it is very expensive to go through
a nurse midwifery training program. When considering it for myself
5 years ago I was a college undergraduate majoring in anthropology.
There was one point then when the homebirths were increasing at such
a rate that I was out doing ten a month myself and sometimes 15. I
couldn't continue school. So at the end of my third year of college,
I didn't know what I wanted to do with my education anyway, and so
I decided I would come back the next year and look for a midwifery
program. Well, I came up with the same thing that many others have
come up with--which was nothing. Despite the three years of college
that I had had, I could not find anything other than going into an
RN program that would require me 4 more years and, at the least, 3
more years of school and then, following that, I would have to go to
a midwifery program which would give me, maybe, a Masters Degree.

By then I had delivered 200 babies and thought, "Well, what the heck. You know, I don't need to go into a Masters Degree program to find out a lot of what I already know." I mean, I would be glad to have the opportunity now to go into a program, but I'd like to be able to go into a program that I see as being reasonable. I just don't believe we need to have five or six years of nursing and midwifery training to become competent midwives.

THERE ARE PROFESSIONALS WHO DO NOT OBJECT TO HOMEBIRTHS BECAUSE THEY FEEL THEM TO BE UNSAFE; THEY OBJECT BECAUSE THEY FEEL THAT HOMEBIRTHS ARE AN "UNECONOMICAL" USE OF THEIR PROFESSIONAL TIME. MY RESPONSE TO THAT IS THAT OUR CONCERN FOR MONEY SEEMS TO BE GREATER THAN OUR CONCERN FOR QUALITY OF CARE.

In California, right now, there is a Bill in the Legislature, Assembly Bill 4492, which is designed to set up a program to study lay midwifery and homebirth. I am looking forward to being involved on that committee considering that bill. There will be obstetricians, nurses, nurse midwives, and lay practitioners on this committee. We are hoping to take back to the State some information that will support the training program being proposed. There is nothing right now. The only training program California had was down near Los Angeles and it closed down last year, unfortunately, because it had to send everyone out of the State to get their "residency" experience. They couldn't do it in the State because, at the time, it was illegal.

Here is my idea of a midwife training program: I would suggest that a two year program, similar to a 2 year RN degree program, is what we need for a midwife. In nurse training programs, there are always prerequisites. Prerequisites for the midwife program could be like one year of liberal arts background, including the sciences that you need, followed by the two years of actual midwifery training. The first six months to a year of the midwife program could stress the important elements of nursing, but the rest of the time should be spent strictly on the midwifery training. Maybe following the training, perhaps the last year, there would be on-the-job training where you would also get paid. Hopefully, a program of this type, which is what I hope we will be able to suggest to this legislative committee, would require a total of three years of schooling with nothing required other than, maybe, the completion of high school prior to getting into the program. Hopefully, completion of such training would result in State Certification or Licensing.

I JUST DON'T BELIEVE WE NEED TO HAVE FIVE OR SIX YEARS OF NURSING AND MIDWIFERY TRAINING TO BECOME COMPETENT MIDWIVES. TWO WEEKS AGO, I RECEIVED TWO LETTERS OF ACCEPTANCE TO TWO SCHOOLS OF NURSING AND I HAVE DECIDED TO TURN THEM BOTH DOWN.

I am very strongly in favor of a training program. I have seen a lot of midwives now in California popping up all over the place. I am very sympathetic because of the way I began and I know of the need. The demand is very, very great. But at the same time, I am very concerned about people going out and attending births, not having any prior training. I don't know if I was just lucky or just blessed in the beginning of my experience. But it concerns me a great deal that somebody might go out and call themselves a midwife and maybe have attended only one birth, or maybe even no births, and then come up with a problem that could really do some damage to a mother or to a baby. So I have to say that I do recognize how important training is and only hope that in the very near future we get some because it will be the only way we are going to be able to meet the needs.

I am very respectful of nurse midwives. I have worked with many of them in California. I think they are making very, very great strides in the hospitals in terms of making beneficial changes. But they won't go out and do homebirths and homebirths aren't going to go away. So what we really need is an alternative midwifery program.

I really see my role as a patient advocate. I think that staying involved with the home and not becoming an obstetrician is really important. Some of the nurse midwives that I have worked with have said, "I wouldn't know what to do if the doctor wasn't there." I think that it's great to have doctor backup but I really don't see a great need to have them in the home. Some of the doctors that I've worked with, though, are great midwives and I'd like to see them continue. I guess more than any learning you could ever get in a school or an institution is learning that you get from the women themselves just by helping them, just being around, listening to them, asking them how they feel.

I do a postpartum visit on the first day. I do a postpartum visit again on the third day and do a PKU test and check the baby to make sure that there is no jaundice. I check again on the second week postpartum mostly to talk about how the family is adjusting to the new baby. One question I always ask is how did you *feel* about the birth and how did you *feel* about me and my part in it. Oftentimes families who are feeling a little concerned or don't understand the procedure that you did or may be just dissatisfied with something that you did will come out and tell you if you give them a chance. I think it is important that we *encourage* families to criticize us so that we can learn better how to help them.

I am in midwifery because of my great concern, not for homebirth, but for birth. Homebirth is really a lovely thing. But I don't believe the experience of birth has to occur at home. I don't think it has to be at home in order to be a good experience. I've seen women give birth both in the hospital and in the maternity home setting have a beautiful experience. All of you women out there who have pushed out a baby, you weren't looking at what was on the walls when you were pushing that baby out. The beauty and the joy that you get from giving birth doesn't come from the location that you are in.

Birth consists of relationships between people. In midwifery the thing that I have gotten through my experiences is really a very profound respect for what goes on, how people relate to each other, and the need for children to be present when their mother gives birth. When my third child was born, my daughters were in school in the second and third grades. I was anxious for them to get home because I couldn't imagine giving birth before they came in from school. They knew that baby was in me all the time, but I just didn't know how I would be able to tell them how it came out. And so, to have them there to be able to see it was really important for me.

I THINK IT IS IMPORTANT THAT WE WHO ATTEND BIRTHS ENCOURAGE FAMILIES TO CRITICIZE US SO THAT WE CAN LEARN BETTER HOW TO HELP THEM.

Through the years I think the things that I have seen have helped me learn how to help women deliver their own babies and have a more satisfying experience in doing so. One time, I put my hands in my pockets at a birth. I said, "the only way I'm going to learn how to not interfere with birth is to keep my hands out of it." And I did it and it scared the hell out of me. But it turns out, there were no problems. That baby and mother did just fine.

The thing that I am doing now at homebirth is having ladies sit up and initially touch the baby's head when it is crowning. It has taken a long time for me to get to a place where I feel comfortable doing it myself. It's amazing the resistance I get at the elbow when I try to pull a woman's arm down and get her to touch the head of that baby. But you ought to see her face when she does it. It's fantastic what happens to her. I have heard women say to me, "Thank you for letting me touch my baby as it was coming out." One woman who had her hand on that head as it emerged said to me the next day, "You know, I felt one with myself. I felt I was giving birth to myself and my baby. It was one of the most wonderful things that ever happened to me." I think the level of satisfaction for women to participate in their birth is just amazing.

BIRTH CONSISTS OF RELATIONSHIPS BETWEEN PEOPLE.

One lady's mother came along to the birth. She sat for hours and hours and hours helping her daughter, stroking her forehead with a cool washrag. When that baby was born there were tears in that mother's eyes and she turned to her daughter and said, "I envy you."

ONE OF THE THINGS I DO OVER AND OVER AGAIN AT A BIRTH WHERE THERE ARE CHILDREN IS GRIN AT THE KIDS A LOT. IT KEEPS THEM REALLY HAPPY, CONFIDENT, AND COMFORTABLE.

In the town of Sonoma is a very large community of Jehovah's Witnesses. I have delivered babies at home from them for six years now and continually am called by members of the several churches over there.

ONE TIME I PUT MY HANDS IN MY POCKETS AT A BIRTH. I SAID, "THE ONLY WAY I'M GOING TO LEARN HOW TO NOT INTERFERE WITH BIRTH IS TO KEEP MY HANDS OUT OF IT." AND I DID IT AND IT SCARED THE HELL OUT OF ME. BUT THAT BABY AND MOTHER DID JUST FINE.

In one particular case, with the children present, there was Rachael, four years old, who sat next to her mother the entire time. One of the things that I do over and over again at a birth where there are children is grin at the kids a lot. It keeps them really happy, confident, and comfortable. When Rachael's mother was in hard labor and looking with a stressed look on her face, she reached over to her mother and patted her on the shoulder and said, "Its okay, mommy."

During that birth, Rachael's 15 year old brother had never seen his mother undressed before and was pacing out in the hall when the baby was coming. He was a very sensitive boy, very intelligent. I had been to the home several times and had talked with him. So I kind of knew how he was feeling. I was kind of concerned about him pacing in the hall out there in the middle of the night. So I suggested that he come in and hold the mirror. He hesitated, but then he came in. He watched in awe as his mother gave birth. I looked up when the baby was born and he had tears in his eyes.

After the baby was born, Rachael held the baby first while her brother watched from a distance. He stayed away for a little while. After a few moments he crept closer. Then a little closer. Pretty soon he started criticizing his sister about the way she was holding and caring for the baby. Then he got his hands on the baby. After that, I'll tell you, that mother had a real fight on her hands with both of those children wanting to take care of the baby.

The father, in this instance, was from Austria and had a little mixed emotions about being present at the birth, but he did a fantastic job. And the second that baby was born he was out in the kitchen and cooked us up a great dinner.

There is an interesting thing about infant bonding illustrated in this experience with the two children. Marshall Klaus has been doing studies on mother-infant bonding and we have been helping with photographs. At one birth, Suzanne Arms and I must have taken a picture every 10 seconds throughout the whole labor. What Dr. Klaus is looking for are "species specific" behavior patterns that come out so beautifully in homebirths, unperturbed by the hospital. In fact he said to me, "You know, Nancy, I loved the pictures you sent me of homebirths. I think I want to come out to California and see some because I now realize that there is no good way to really study this whole thing of bonding when I have never seen normal birth where it belongs--in the home." Now the thing that has been discovered lately is that humans, when they first pick up a newborn, will take one finger and stroke the baby's cheek. They do it over and over again. We have seen this time and time again with mothers.

But the interesting thing is that when this 15 year old boy was first holding that newborn baby I found him cuddling, looking, and with his finger out there touching that baby's cheek the very same way women do.

I will conclude by saying that I really see my role now as helping women to help themselves. Watching women give birth and helping them to deliver their own babies has just been fantastic for me. It has taken a real evolution for me to learn how to help women help themselves and have a satisfying experience. And I am really happy to see that it is possible. I think it can be possible wherever you have good support for women--either in a hospital or in a home. I just hope that the law permits us to continue.

And one final thing for all you ladies out there who are interested in midwifery: Two weeks ago I received two letters of acceptance to two schools of nursing in California. I have decided to turn them both down.

Why Do Responsible, Informed Parents Choose Homebirths?
(FOUR ESSAYS BY PARENTS OPTING FOR BIRTH AT HOME)

1. CUSTOM-MADE DELIVERY
   by Marian Tompson, Franklin Park, IL
2. HOMEBIRTH: A FAMILY AWAKENING
   by Cedar & Stephen Koons, Hillsborough, NC
3. BIRTH IN A GROCERY STORE
   by Hart & Neil Collins, Raleigh, NC
4. CONTROL IS THE KEY
   By Martha & William Longbrake, College Park, MD

* *

1. Custom-Made Delivery
Marian Tompson*

It never occurred to me when expecting my first baby that I would ever want to have a baby at home. All I wanted then was natural childbirth. Years before, in high school, I had read an article about Grantly Dick-Read which made so much sense that as soon as I became pregnant the first thing I did was to go to the bookstore and purchase "Childbirth Without Fear". In total naivete, I told my obstetrician that this was how I wanted to deliver my baby and, although he had never delivered an undrugged lady before, he agreed to go along with me and let me have my baby without drugs or anesthetics. And do you know, he actually did!

My first labor, though, was 36 hours long because the baby was posterior, and the doctor was a little unhappy because, as he reminded me, if I was knocked out he could just slip in those forceps and have that baby out in a minute. The actual delivery was painless and one of the most exciting moments of my life.

Because I was awake during labor I became most aware of how unsuitable a place a hospital is in which to have a baby, and how insensitive many birth attendants are to the needs of the woman in labor. There was the night nurse who insisted on turning off the lights in the labor room as I approached transition because "it's night-time now and you should go to sleep." And the day nurse who asserted that "the Read method is fine in theory, but it won't work once you get in the delivery room."

One of the most dismaying things to me about the whole experience was when I went to the hospital, I was so excited. "This is going to be the birthday of my baby!" I kept thinking. And yet nobody there was excited about it at all. I could have been going to have my toenails cut for all they cared. I would have loved one

---

* MARIAN TOMPSON is a Founding Mother and President of La Leche League International; she and her husband, Clement, are parents of seven children, the last four at home attended by Gregory White, MD; Clement is an Electrical Engineer with his own Electronic Systems Consulting Business in Chicago.

person to say, "Gee, you know, isn't this wonderful. You're going to have your baby today." How I would have appreciated just one acknowledgement that this was really a special day for me, just one person who understood and shared my excitement at what was taking place.

There were two beds in the labor room, which was right next to the delivery room, and my husband had to take turns being in the room with the other occupant's husband. If someone was in the delivery toom, both husbands were kept out of the labor room. Husbands were NOT allowed in the delivery room.

So you can understand why, for my next two deliveries, I delayed going to the hospital until the last minute. The only thing I didn't like about having a baby was *where* I had to have it.

There was also some confusion in the hospital as to just who delivered the baby. This was well illustrated when I arrived at the hospital for my second delivery the following year. I had asked my doctor if my husband could be with me in the delivery room this time. He said, "Oh, no. This just isn't allowed and anyway, *there wouldn't be room.*" I really didn't understand that. You see, natural childbirth wasn't too common 25 years ago and unbeknownst to me, a number of physicians, externs, interns, and clerks had asked to be allowed to be in the delivery room to view the event. Unfortunately, my doctor's office nurse also wanted to be included. This caused a problem because when I arrived at the hospital so close to delivery, having waited until the last minute, the doctor was in his office and had to wait for his nurse to close down the office so he could drive her to the hospital to see my birth. Even though I was almost ready to have my baby, the other doctors there on call were afraid to do anything to me because they didn't want to mess up this unusual happening. So I was wheeled right into the delivery room, asked to please keep my legs together and not to bear down, and then left alone. When my doctor arrived it reminded me of those triumphal processions where the king enters the captured city. All it really lacked was the bugles. First came a nurse walking backwards, the better to put his gloves on, and directly in back of him another nurse, tying up his gown. Behind them, the spectators, who quickly filled the room. "Doctor, they won't let me push," I said. "Marian, you can push now," he said. So with three pushes, no tearing, and no screaming my beautiful dark-haired Deborah was born. And as I joyfully reached out to touch her, one of the residents rushed up to my physician and said, "Doctor, how did you do it?"

THE DOCTOR SAID, "MARIAN, YOU CAN PUSH NOW." SO WITH THREE PUSHES, NO TEARING, AND NO SCREAMING MY BEAUTIFUL DARK-HAIRED DEBORAH WAS BORN. AND AS I JOYFULLY REACHED OUT TO TOUCH HER, ONE OF THE RESIDENTS RUSHED UP TO MY PHYSICIAN AND SAID, "DOCTOR, HOW DID YOU DO IT!"

You can imagine my elation upon discovering that Dr. Gregory White, a local doctor, actually allowed mothers to deliver their babies at home. So with my fourth pregnancy we made plans for a homebirth. At first my husband was understandably concerned about safety, but after reading a few studies on home versus hospital deliveries he realized the odds were in our favor in most ways, and after we had that first homebirth he would never even consider any other way. One of my great joys during that birth was watching the wonder on his face as our fourth daughter was born. After that we had a fifth daughter and two sons--four homebirths in all.

Homebirths were for me custom-made deliveries. During labor I was no longer confined to a small room but could sit or walk around inside or out of the house. There was none of that apprehension I felt in the hospital when strange people, calling me "mother", came in and poked and prodded, but never could tell me what was going on because "only the doctor could do that." I had found it frightening in the hospital to be alone and at the mercy of strangers during such a crucial time. At home we could make most of the decisions, including who would be present. My husband was with me, both for the support which I needed and to share the awe-filled event. No one could take my baby away from me at a time when we both needed each other. And while our other children were never in the room during the delivery they usually were there minutes afterwards. Then, after tying an appropriately colored delivery blanket to the lamp post outside to share the good news with our neighbors, we would celebrate with a small birthday party. Breastfeeding proceeded on demand following the baby's need and with a minimum of engorgement.

I know it's not fashionable to talk about things that can't be measured scientifically, yet many of the advantages of homebirth belong in that category. Unless they've experienced it you can't expect people to understand what it means to give birth to a baby in your own bed, surrounded only by people who love and care about you, and to be in a position to truly celebrate a birth rather than just bravely endure it. The effects of these unmeasurables should not be underestimated.

After that first hospital delivery, I seriously considered becoming a midwife after my children were grown or, failing that, hoped that maybe I could just go sit in labor rooms helping to make birth a more positive experience for other women. Well, in an unexpected and beautiful way, that second wish sort of came true last Fall when our daughter, Deborah, and her husband, Wayne, decided to have their first baby, and our first grandchild, at home. Michelle's birth was attended by her father, by Dr. William White, son of Gregory White, and by this lucky grandmother. But that's another whole story and maybe someday I'll have an opportunity to tell you about it.

2. HOMEBIRTH: A FAMILY AWAKENING

Cedar Koons & Stephen Koons*

CEDAR: We chose to have our baby at home because we wanted to
experience birth in an atmosphere of love and respect for what we
consider to be a miracle--the beginning of life. Early in my pregnancy we felt that at home, surrounded by the people that we chose,
we could share what was to us a kind of "rite of passage" into
parenthood in the same spirit that we shared our marriage. When we
got married we didn't go to the Justice of the Peace and stand in
line with a lot of other couples. Some people may do that and
that's fine. But what we did was go out into the woods with a
group of our friends and at daybreak, at 7:00 in the morning, we
got married. So when it came time to have our baby, it just didn't
seem like what we wanted to do, to go into a hospital labor room
and wait on the assembly line until it was time to go to the delivery room and then be ushered out and upstairs to the postpartum
maternity ward.

We knew that in order for our choice to be a responsible one
necessitated tremendous preparation. We knew that it was a real
responsibility and we deeply felt that responsibility for the child
we had conceived. We conceived the child without medical help. I
carried it in my body and nourished it as it grew--all by natural,
nonmedical means. We decided we wanted to give birth in the same
natural way. We knew other people could help us but only we could
really discharge the full responsibility and we knew this would be
so whether in the hospital or in the home. So we saw this tremendous preparation ahead of us and we took it on with joy.

I have always been a healthy person. I try to be attentive to
my diet and see to the need for wholesome foods and a balanced kind
of simple life--as simple as the 20th Century allows. I see that
true health begins in one's consciousness, that the health of the
body and the health of the spirit go hand in hand. So when I became pregnant, I looked forward to a normal, nine months of inten-
sified consciousness, culminating in a normal, natural labor. I
expected it to be strenuous. I expected it to be hard work, but I
expected it to be a natural thing that I could handle. I had full
faith that my body, given its health and good diet with adequate
prenatal medical care, would function as it was created to do.

---

* CEDAR & STEPHEN KOONS *are cofounders and officers of NAPSAC,
Stephen being Treasurer and Cedar being NAPSAC News Editor; the Koons
own their own business, the Rainbow Water Service, that distributes
bottled water. They also teach homebirth preparation classes and are
involved in organizing local groups to establish safe homebirth programs. They are the parents of one child, born at home, attended by
a Physician's Associate--a friend of theirs.*

I went through all the doubts in my mind. I went through all of the fears. I went through the whole dark night of the soul. You know the sorts of things I mean: "What if the baby doesn't breathe?" "What if this or that?" I was never really worried about whether I would hemorrhage. That was just one particular thing I wasn't worried about. And at one point my obstetrician said, "You know, have you ever thought that you could stop yourself bleeding by just thinking about it?" I thought, "Golly, this coming from an obstetrician is pretty strange." But, you know, I do think there is something to one's consciousness having control over the material aspects. Certainly, you can at least control your reactions to things. And by being calm, you can handle any situation better.

I HAD FULL FAITH THAT MY BODY, GIVEN ITS HEALTH AND GOOD DIET WITH ADEQUATE PRENATAL MEDICAL CARE, WOULD FUNCTION AS IT WAS CREATED TO DO.

I never expected to have my baby in the hospital even though I understood there is a time should nature fail when the hospital is the best and the proper place for birth. I had shared a homebirth of a friend and found it to be a wonderful experience. But even before that, before I was pregnant, before I ever saw a birth at home, I never wanted to be delivered in a hospital. I spent one stay in the hospital when I was 11 years old and found it to be a very unpleasant place. And maybe my dislike for hospitals goes back to feminism, where in some of my gynecological and obstetrical experiences in a hospital I felt that I was not given the full respect that I was due as a human being. And then I am just the kind of person who would rather do it herself. One thing I wanted very much was to be in control of the birthing energy that was around me and I couldn't feel that once I went into that big institution that I would have that control. Hospitals are pervaded with sickness, the risk of intervention, unnatural practices, strange procedures, strange rules, strange food, no natural lighting--all of those things just didn't seem the right place for me to have a baby.

I also wanted Stephen to catch the baby. Stephen is my husband. Our birth was attended by a physician's associate, a PA. He was a friend of ours and we wanted him there. He is a wonderful person and was willing to come. It was comfortable to have him there and yet he wasn't really there--that is, he didn't really deliver my baby. His support was there but all he did was kind of say, "Uh,huh. Yes. Okay. Everything's fine," and reassuring things like that and it was good to have him there. But Stephen, my husband, caught the baby because we feel that birth is a deeply intimate act of love. It is something beyond conception. It is something that I think every woman should be able to share with someone in that bonding of love, experiencing and sharing with someone else the birth of her child. For me that someone was my husband.

A most important consideration was that I did not want to be separated from my baby and I did not want Stephen to be separated from me and his newborn child. When I did give cursory thought to having a baby in the hospital, that was the cutoff point. I knew that if they came and wanted to take my baby to the nursery right after birth I was going to have a screaming fit. I just didn't want to go through that after I had had a baby. So I decided to stay home because all the hospitals in our area routinely separate mothers and babies in those crucial hours. Anybody who has had a baby nestled in their own bed and was able to marvel at their new-born would know and understand why having the baby with you is such a precious thing.

WHEN I DID GIVE CURSORY THOUGHT TO HAVING THE BABY IN THE HOSPITAL, THE THOUGHT OF HAVING THE BABY TAKEN FROM ME AND PUT IN A NURSERY WAS THE CUTOFF POINT. I KNEW I WOULD HAVE A SCREAMING FIT IF THEY TRIED TO DO THAT AND I JUST DIDN'T WANT TO HAVE TO GO THROUGH THAT. SO I STAYED HOME.

In our area, we have no homebirth program. We don't have nurse midwives or lay midwives who will deliver at home. The official policy is opposed to homebirths. I got a tremendous amount of negative energy from various professionals to whom I went for prenatal assistance. Eventually, I found good prenatal care from a sympathetic doctor.

Finally, we had to trust our own good judgement. I think that people are often too unwilling to trust in their own judgement. I think it is essential for responsible adults to be able to say, "Okay, I have gotten as much information as I can get. I have talked to people. I've read. I've thought about it. Now I am going to trust my judgement." As a couple, we felt that we knew the signs of possible complications and should any of them appear during labor, we would have gone into the hospital.

Our daughter, Woodwyn Whiteoak, was born seven months ago today. Everything was very straightforward. It was a wonderful experience. Both Stephen and I feel that the joy of her birth, being able to assume the role as parents from the beginning, the absence of the interference of imposed routine, and the simple sur-rounding beauty of our home at birth have provided us with the firmest foundation for our parenthood.

STEPHEN: We live down in North Carolina on a farm. It's kind of a simple life. This is one of the things that I think really exercises a strong influence upon me as both a parent and as a person. If we can just simplify our life even a little tiny bit, there's such an inpouring of beauty and richness that had gone un-noticed before. There's a real truer awareness of who we are and what our relationship to our universe is. Simplicity can grant us a glimpse of a world in harmony that's sensitive to the needs of everybody. Simplicity is kind of like nature at work. In order to enjoy the rewards of nature, we have to be open participants in it. I guess that's really why we chose homebirth, because we wanted to enjoy the experience of creation happening right before our eyes and to be able to share that with others.

There is so much beauty in birth that it is very difficult to put into words. It's kind of hard to talk about why we made the choice of a homebirth because it is like that choice was made a long time ago--back before there were hospitals and back before there were doctors. It was a very natural thing to us. We wanted to consciously attend to the growth of the new life that was begun between us and to apply that growth to our capacity to be loving parents. We saw that our family was going to be centered in the home from the point that the baby arrived and it was just natural that we should attend to that happening right there in the home from its very beginning--not wait until the baby came from outside somewhere and then start to get it on at home. So we started at home and made that our first place of focus.

IN ORDER TO ENJOY THE REWARDS OF NATURE, WE HAVE TO BE OPEN PARTICIPANTS IN IT, AND THAT'S REALLY WHY WE CHOSE HOMEBIRTH, BECAUSE WE WANTED TO ENJOY THE EXPERIENCE OF CREATION HAPPENING RIGHT BEFORE OUR EYES.

We conceived our child at home. We pored over books and pictures about birth at home. We talked with friends and between ourselves about birth at home. We sat out on the backporch and watched the stars and the moon slide by at home and, quite simply, it never really occurred to us that the day of birth we had been anticipating with so much joy should happen any place else. That was our starting place to dig in and really see where we were, where our fears were coming from and how to get rid of them.

We made arrangements with a friendly doctor at a local hospital in case our situation should indicate medical intervention. Just having that outpost of trust in the hospital made our confidence and commitment to a truly natural birth a lot greater. But the hospital atmosphere of technology and drugs, of haste and pathological theory didn't seem to have very much bearing on the lessons and rewards of simplicity. We toured the OB ward at the hospital and after that we were sure that we didn't want to have our child come into a group of strangers at such a place but rather into the loving circle of family and friends in a familiar setting. We also felt strongly that our child should emerge into her father's hands and share that first breath of life in the intimate bond of family. We felt then, and we feel very strongly now, that that is one of the most crucial moments in the establishment of a peaceful world because it contains such potential for understanding and realizing what our purpose is here and for assuming the responsibility to that purpose.

WE FEEL THAT BIRTH IS ONE OF THE MOST CRUCIAL MOMENTS IN THE ESTABLISHMENT OF A PEACEFUL WORLD BECAUSE IT CONTAINS SUCH POTENTIAL FOR UNDERSTANDING AND REALIZING WHAT OUR PURPOSE IS HERE AND FOR ASSUMING THE RESPONSIBILITY TO THAT PURPOSE.

We couldn't have done this by ourselves. There are really a lot of factors that allowed us to realize our choice of homebirth. I will just briefly mention three of them. First of all is the love that our parents gave to us as their children so that we could see ourselves as being responsible parents in turn. It's kind of like that picture painted by Michelangelo where the guy is lying there with his one hand up and his other down and somebody is about to touch it up here. It's like being a part of that circle.

Secondly, early in our pregnancy we had been present at the birth of the son of our two good friends, John and Mickey Jo. Their boy, Seth, was born in a cozy cabin with a fire on the hearth and it was one of the most beautiful experiences I had ever had because we had witnessed creation directly and had found it full and complete and we just sank roots down into that experience and started building for our own child's birth yet to come.

Thirdly, we had support and knowledge and experience of a loving community of people who were really committed to truly natural birth.

Each factor played its vital part in the good experience we had in birth. With that good beginning, all we can do now is grow and I am very happy about that.

IF WE CAN JUST SIMPLIFY OUR LIFE EVEN A LITTLE TINY BIT, THERE'S SUCH AN INPOURING OF BEAUTY AND RICHNESS THAT HAD GONE UNNOTICED BEFORE.

---

3. BIRTH IN A GROCERY STORE

Hart Collins & Neil Collins, JD*

NEIL: Three months ago I helped my wife give birth to our second daughter. No doctor was there. We had not planned on one. Nor was a midwife there. We had decided about 2 weeks before the birth that if the midwife wasn't there, we could still manage. As the baby was about to be born, the only thing I was worried about was keeping my wife in good spirits. Over the past six months my thoughts had evolved from "Of course not!" through "I hope not!" into "Oh dear!" to "Sure" and finally to "I can." We had come to the conclusion that the safety factor in a homebirth was, in our case, equal to that of a hospital birth. And we had even decided that for us it was not essential to have an attendant, that if the presence of a midwife were that critical then we wouldn't be choosing a homebirth.

I wasn't worried at all when it started back when my wife first said she wanted a homebirth. I assumed she would see the light of reasonableness and change her mind. That was when she was 3 months' pregnant. When she was 4 months'pregnant and said the same thing, I began to get worried. I didn't know too many facts about homebirth. I did know that as an attorney when you told a client, "there probably won't be any problems," that such statements are always qualified by 37 clauses each starting with "if" or "so long as."

The logical corollary was that hospitals and obstetricians didn't just *happen* to be in the business of delivering babies. Society relies on professions--in some cases with very good cause. What could be more important, and therefore in need of more professional care, than a birth? That was my major problem in the beginning.

The only reason I went along was because I also assumed that if a homebirth were actually a reasonable alternative to a hospital, then there must be some competent doctor who would help out at our homebirth--albeit on the sly. And I knew my super-efficient wife would find him or her. Confident in the knowledge that I could be a calm bystander, I kept going to the childbirth classes we were attending at the time.

The first dent in the theory that "the hospital is the only answer" came with the statement that one of the primary reasons that births were first brought into hospitals was because of the use of anesthetics. I didn't like that. I wanted the hospital to be "the answer," but instead it was as though I was being told that a garage mechanic put a radiator on my air-cooled engine and now I needed a checkup on my radiator.

---

* *HART & NEIL COLLINS are parents of two children, the first born in a hospital and the second at home without medical attendance; Hart has completed two years of college with a major in Russian and Neil is an Attorney at Law with the U.S. Environmental Protection Agency, Research Triangle Park, NC, and is the Attorney for NAPSAC.*

THE IMPORTANT THING IS NOT WHETHER HOMEBIRTH IS MORE OR LESS SAFE THAN HOSPITALS. THE IMPORTANT THING IS THAT A REASONABLE FAMILY CAN COME TO SUCH A DECISION. IT THEN BECOMES THE DUTY OF HEALTH PROFESSIONALS TO HELP AS BEST THEY CAN.

Then I said to myself, "What's a hospital good for?" Competent people and emergency equipment, of course. So why not bring a competent attendant to your home and go to the hospital in the case of an emergency. I was still assuming that we would find that competent person to help if the birth was at home. Little did I know that ultimately I would be elected. The next question is: When do you need emergency equipment? For emergencies. When do you have to have heart surgery? I assumed it wasn't too often. I knew that the odds could not possibly be more in favor of my wife and baby. My wife was super healthy--riding a bicycle daily 15 to 20 miles until her stomach got too big and her knees kept bumping it; then jogging a mile and a half nightly up to the night before labor started. She had a super diet: considerably over the recommended protein intake for pregnant ladies, and she's small. Besides we knew she had a body that could birth a child. We already had one. And she had an obstetrician whose competence was cross-referenced from several other health professionals who, themselves, had reputations for excellence.

The obstetrician knew my wife was going to have a homebirth. He said things looked OK, and that the baby wasn't early or late, etc., and he wasn't worried. Now that worried me. I knew I was getting drawn into the active planning for a homebirth. I started practicing infant artificial resuscitation by timing my blowing into my fist (I didn't tell my wife).

I WASN'T WORRIED AT ALL WHEN MY WIFE FIRST SAID SHE WANTED A HOMEBIRTH EARLY IN HER PREGNANCY. I ASSUMED SHE WOULD SEE THE LIGHT OF REASONABLENESS AND CHANGE HER MIND.

My decision that a homebirth could be safe need not be judged for the truth that may or may not underlie it. What is important is that a reasonable family can come to such a decision. And if a reasonable family, one no different from many others by all external evidence, can make that decision then health professionals have a duty to assist as best they can.

But the nice part about our deciding that a homebirth could be safe was that it allowed me to release some primal emotions and think in terms of "wouldn't it be nice if we could have our baby in our own bedroom." As birth became imminent we became more and more certain that we didn't want our baby to be born in a place that seemed no more appropriate than a birth in a grocery store. Full of strange sounds, and sights, and coldness. It's enough to make you cry. And then the people poking, shoving, giving orders, or maybe even a sweet smile, but just when you wanted to be alone.

The birth of my baby is a sacred family event and should be treated as such. We need quiet, time alone, familiar surroundings while we undergo the world's stress of a new creation--it is not a time to be in a grocery store.

HART: Four years ago when I was pregnant for the first time, I thought all babies were born in hospitals. However, when Neil and I were taking childbirth preparation classes back then when we lived in Washington, DC, another of the mothers-to-be in that class was planning to deliver at home with Dr. Brew. The idea was immediately appealing to me. It intuitively seemed right to give birth in the comfort of my own bedroom. But I also knew I was not prepared, and besides, when I asked my OB to deliver at our home, he declined. I thought that with 7 weeks to go, I was too far into the pregnancy to change doctors.

We went ahead with the planned hospital delivery and were only too glad to get out of the hospital within twelve hours afterwards. I relived the experience for weeks afterwards--disappointed in myself for not refusing the Demerol and insisting on keeping the baby with me. My labor had totaled 23 hours and I was certain my alienation by the hospital atmosphere had prolonged the birth process. That hospital experience did have value, however, because it served to dispel a lifetime's accumulated misconceptions about childbirth, doctors, and hospitals.

CHILDBIRTH HAD NOT BEEN EXPERIENCED BY ME THE FIRST TIME AS A DANGEROUS OR FEARFUL THING - IT WAS THE DISRUPTIVE HOSPITAL ROUTINES THAT HAD CAUSED THE TRAUMA.

In the meantime, we moved to North Carolina. So when I became pregnant again one year ago, I began to search people and books to tell me more about homebirths. First, I set about finding a doctor in North Carolina who, like Dr. Brew in Washington, would come to our home. I was surprised by the opposition I encountered. The first doctor I consulted no longer supported home deliveries, saying that he felt the infant "deserved" the safety of a hospital birth. I knew my resolution to have the baby at home would fail if I could not find a supportive doctor. Fortunately, the second one I consulted was very reassuring about answering all of my "what if" questions. He predicted we would encounter no problems if I maintained good prenatal care. None of his homebirth patients had had a bad experience, he told me.

Finding a supportive doctor was only the first hurdle. Since my doctor would not come to our home, our next problem was to find a medical attendant. Early in my pregnancy I considered an attendant an absolute prerequisite for a safe homebirth. So I spent my first two trimesters calling every possible lead trying to locate a medical attendant--nurse, paramedic, physician's associate, nurse practitioner. But I could find no one who would risk breaking the law, even though I explained they could come in a nonmedical capacity.

Meanwhile, we had been preparing ourselves for the homebirth. We understood that something like 95% of the risks could be prevented by excellent prenatal care, so I had tried to eat 100 grams of complete protein per day and also maintained an aerobics program of bicycling and jogging. From the 4th month on, we had attended childbirth preparation classes geared particularly for homebirth parents and we read our way through a library of childbirth books.

I WAS ANNOYED WITH THE MEDICAL ESTABLISHMENT FOR GIVING US THE UNSPOKEN ULTIMATUM - "EITHER YOU COME TO THE HOSPITAL AND BE SAFE OR STAY HOME AND TAKE YOUR CHANCES."

My anticipation of the homebirth grew with the baby inside me. I was eager to experience an intimate family birth with my husband catching the baby, rather than observing as a passive bystander. I wanted my three year old daughter to witness the birth and gain a firsthand understanding of "Where do babies come from?" I couldn't wait to lie in bed with my new infant, touching, reveling in each other without anxiety over imminent separation. I looked forward to sleeping after the birth with my child and my husband beside me in our own bed, not in a strange place surrounded by strangers. I wanted to be able to fully relax during my labor in pleasant surroundings, and not be monitored, poked, inspected, or probed. I simply wanted too much from the birth experience to settle for another hospital birth. Our baby "deserved" a lot more than what hospitals could offer.

WE REALIZED THAT SOCIETY WOULD TRY TO HANG A HEAVY BURDEN OF GUILT ON US IF OUR HOMEBIRTH WERE TO END TRAGICALLY. BUT THE MORE I READ, THE LESS RESPONSIBLE IT SEEMED TO SUBJECT AN INFANT TO A HOSPITAL.

I was entering my last trimester before I finally realized that there really was no one to attend our birth. So we had to choose whether to drop the whole idea or to go ahead on our own. I had done too much reading and soul searching in preparation for the homebirth by this time to be able to just drop the idea and embrace a hospital birth. My stubbornness may have become a factor here.

WE BEGAN TO PERCEIVE THE HOSPITAL AS MERELY AN EXCUSE TO PIN THE GUILTY LABEL ON SOMEONE ELSE FOR AN UNHAPPY EXPERIENCE.

I was annoyed with the medical establishment for giving us the unspoken ultimatum - "Either you come to the hospital and be safe or stay home and take your chances." We realized that society would try to hang a heavy burden of guilt on us if our homebirth were to end tragically. But the more I read, the less responsible it seemed to subject an infant to a hospital birth. The hospital was merely an excuse, it seemed, to pin the guilty label on someone else for an unhappy experience.

I had a gut conviction that since I was a whole, healthy person, my body would give birth in its matter-of-fact fashion to a whole and healthy infant. Childbirth had not been experienced by me the first time as a dangerous or fearful thing - it was the disruptive hospital routines that had caused the trauma. I was not anxious for my own safety since we could easily reach a hospital before I bled to death. As for the infant's safety, I felt convinced that I had eliminated all the risks over which I had control by my conscientious prenatal care. I was not convinced that a hospital birth was a guaranteed safe birth for the infant anyway, although I would not hesitate to use the hospital if complications arose during labor.

IF, AFTER HUNDREDS OF YEARS OF MEDDLING, MEDICINE CANNOT CLAIM TO HAVE ERADICATED THE RISK FROM CHILDBIRTH, PERHAPS THERE WERE NOT MEANT TO BE ANY GUARANTEES IN CHILDBIRTH.

If I sound preoccupied with weighing the risks, it is because I felt considerable pressure from our family and friends to justify a decision that appeared irrational to them. "How can you dare to give birth away from the hospital's lifesaving equipment?" they asked. I could only offer our example as an answer: If, after hundreds of years of meddling, medicine could not claim to have eradicated the risk from childbirth, perhaps there were not meant to be any guarantees in childbirth.

In my 8th month I had this flash of what I took for insight-- that perhaps birth was meant to be a part of creation, the destiny of the infant on its journey from the womb was not meant to be under the jurisdiction of any man or woman. I came to see birth as a part of the love act between man and wife that does not require supervision any more than the act of conception.

In the final weeks of my pregnancy, I was relaxed and thankful that just the two of us would be attending our birth. I was *glad* that we had *not* found an attendant and hoped no one would come forward in the remaining weeks.

With our second child, we simply asserted our responsibility over her well-being beginning with the time of conception, rather than waiting until we walked out of the hospital doors.

4. CONTROL IS THE KEY

Martha Longbrake, RN & William A. Longbrake, DBA*

To be in control of the fantastic event of the birth of our children was the basic reason that we chose homebirth. Yet, when we were first asked "why?" our answer would not have been "control." It was only as we reflected about the events preceding the births of our children, as well as the deliveries themselves, in the process of writing this that we realized the importance of our desire and *need* to be in control.

Because control and some other secondary motivations were not fully apparent to us until we reexamined and discussed our experiences with each other, we feel that a narrative of these experiences is crucial background material to an understanding of why we, as responsible and informed adults, chose homebirth and why we found it a personally satisfying and self-fulfilling alternative. Our narrative is followed by an analysis of our motivations and reasons.

Martha's interest in alternatives in childbirth--in the sense of involving the father and using exercises and breathing instead of medicated hospital deliveries--began when she was a teenager. She doesn't remember whether it was Dick-Read's "Childbirth Without Fear" or Karmel's "Thank You, Dr. Lamaze" that first stimulated her interest. In any event, once introduced to natural childbirth, she became an advocate, even though at the time marriage and childbearing were the farthest things in her mind.

Bill's interest in alternatives in childbirth really did not begin until he met Martha. He had never really given much thought to the subjects of pregnancy and delivery, figuring that when the time came that would be soon enough to worry about the whole matter. But it proved difficult to ignore Martha's contagious enthusiasm, especially when her involvement in the obstetric rotation in nursing school imparted first hand knowledge of the pregnancy and childbirth experiences of others. She remembers it as a "great summer."

Bill liked the idea of husband involvement and participation in this important family event. In principle, he preferred natural childbirth, but was willing to accept Martha's own preferences because she was the one who would be directly affected. He was prepared to be supportive of whatever course Martha might eventually choose. However, in his quiet, serious manner, he did not convey his interest in prepared childbirth with the same enthusiasm as Martha expressed hers.

---

* *MARTHA & WILLIAM LONGBRAKE are parents of two children, the first born at home attended by both a midwife and a physician, the second born at home by midwife only; William is an Economist with the Federal Deposit Insurance Corporation, Washington, DC. The Longbrakes wish to thank Anne Steinmeyer for typing up their manuscript for this presentation.*

Not yet really understanding Bill's genuine acceptance of her attitude, Martha was concerned whether he would be capable of functioning calmly and rationally in the delivery room. She had heard that the principal objection to fathers in the delivery room was because they fainted. So, without telling Bill her true motive, she took him with her father, who is a veterinarian, on a difficult calving case. Her somewhat illogical reasoning was that if he could see a calf delivered by block and tackle without fainting, she wouldn't have to worry about him in the delivery room some day. He came through with flying colors.

It was not until after we were married and moved to Washington, DC, that Martha discovered some who were *not* poor, *not* poorly educated, and *not* hippies who had their babies at home. When Martha's operating room colleague, Judy Melson, talked about having her second baby at home, Martha asked interested questions, all the while thinking back to her OB nursing lectures of the 4% of deliveries that involved complications. She remembers thinking at first that home deliveries might be fine for some, but not for her. However, her feeling that the entire thing bordered on irresponsibility was tempered by her understanding from what Judy had said that she was required to have had a normal hospital delivery *before* her doctor, Dr. Brew, would consider a home delivery.

In retrospect, Martha feels that her only real concern was if medical intervention might be required, the hospital would be the best place to be. She had no difficulty accepting other aspects of home delivery such as the absence of medication, no sterile field, and the lack of an opportunity to rest and recuperate afterward.

Martha chose Dr. Brew as her OB because of his reputation of favoring husband-involved, prepared childbirth. In the course of routine checkups she met many interesting people, some of whom were planning or had had home deliveries. After each visit, Martha enthusiastically recounted her conversations to Bill. Although neither of us was really aware at the time, the stage was being set for facing the decision of home delivery in an informed way later on.

When the decision to begin a family was reached early in 1973, Martha reread all the books on childbirth she had been accumulating and made special trips to the bookstore and the library to acquire ones she had not read. Bill didn't need to read much because Martha filled him in on the details and even read especially interesting passages out loud. Both of us agreed that prepared childbirth was the way we wanted to do things, if at all possible.

Finally, Martha was pregnant. It was accepted as a matter of course that we would attend childbirth education classes, that Bill would be totally involved, that Martha would breastfeed, and that we would choose a hospital that provided rooming-in accommodations. Both of us had visited friends that chose rooming-in and we were both impressed by how this enabled the family to be close right from the beginning. Furthermore, this arrangement strives to make matters easier for the mother who wishes to breastfeed, another important consideration insofar as we were concerned.

Although we talked a little about homebirth, it was never con-
templated as a feasible alternative. So far as we were aware, the
only doctor who would attend home deliveries would not do it for
first-time mothers. So convinced were we of the reasonableness of
this restriction that Martha in all her visits with Dr. Brew never
once thought of asking him about home deliveries.

MARTHA WAS CONCERNED ABOUT BILL'S POSSIBLY FAINTING AT BIRTH
SO, WITHOUT TELLING HIM HER MOTIVE, SHE ARRANGED FOR HIM TO
ACCOMPANY HER FATHER, WHO WAS A VET, ON A DIFFICULT DELIVERY OF A
CALF ON THE THEORY THAT IF BILL COULD MAKE IT THRU A BOVINE BIRTH
BY BLOCK & TACKLE WITHOUT FAINTING, HE WOULD SURELY THEN BE PREPARED
FOR FOR A HUMAN BIRTH THAT WAS NORMAL.

It wasn't until the evening when Bill accompanied Martha to
Dr. Brew's office for the first time that we decided to ask him. We
were chatting with a young couple who were also expecting their
first child while waiting for our turn when another patient said to
the young couple, "I see you brought your map with you." "What in
the world!" thought Martha. It was a map to their house--for a home
delivery! Surprised, Martha's immediate response was, "But I thought
he didn't do it at home unless you'd had one normal hospital delivery." We were assured that this was, in fact, their first; they had
just recently moved to Washington from California and had sought out
Dr. Brew purposely. In California they had been planning to have a
home delivery without a physician in attendance. As we waited, we
asked a lot of questions. Martha did most of the talking and Bill
could see the sparkle in her eyes and sensed the excitement in her
voice. Knowing that Martha's curiosity and interest had been
aroused, Bill suggested, "Why don't you ask Dr. Brew about your having a home delivery. This is your chance to do it."

Martha recalls that this was said so coolly and seriously it
was just as if we had discussed it at length and had decided homebirth was for us. Up until this time, Martha had really expected to
have *all* her children in the hospital. However, if Bill was so sure
a home delivery was what we wanted, Martha reasoned, she wasn't
about to be against it. She remembers this evening as one in which
a momentous decision was made naturally with no premeditation.

Bill says that this impression is not accurate. We were prepared. We had done considerable background reading. We had talked
about the subject at length, though not in reference to ourselves.
So when the opportunity presented itself, we could make what we felt
to be a "natural" choice. Bill also says that he assumed Martha was
interested in the subject. He's right about the first part--it
wasn't just a spur-of-the-moment decision, however spontaneous it
may have seemed. But as to the second part, Martha says that she
truly never considered home delivery seriously for herself until
Bill expressed such obvious favor for the idea and suggested, that
evening, that we should ask Dr. Brew about it.

A seemingly natural decision, yet, there were questions. What if something happened? To Martha? We had faith that Dr. Brew would know ahead of time if there were likely to be problems. And, as unrealistic as it might sound, we couldn't conceive of anything happening that would cause dire consequences before Martha could get to the nearest hospital three miles away.

What if something happened to the baby? This one was harder. However, Martha knew from her nurse's training that if the baby had a problem requiring heroic measures for survival and couldn't live until we could get help, there was serious question about the quality of life he would have. Off setting this concern, we believed that a natural, nonmedicated birth in comfortable, quiet surroundings would give the baby the best possible introduction into his new world.

Then there were parents, friends, and neighbors to consider. Over the long-distance lines we announced to Martha's father that we were going to have his first grandchild at home. "Don't be ridiculous!" he responded in the same tone you would reply to your eight-year-old who had just told you he was going to spend a cold rainy December night sleeping in his friend's backyard trying out a new tent. Living nearly 1,000 miles distant from Martha's parents, we didn't mention homebirth again until we sent pictures of grandson number one's delivery.

AT HOME, INSTEAD OF US BEING INTRUDERS INTO THE WORLD OF THE MEDICAL PERSONNEL, THE MIDWIFE AND THE DOCTOR WOULD BE VISITORS.

Fortunately, Bill's parents, especially his mother, expressed interest. His mother said she would come to help out and, of course, we invited her to be present at the birth. Arrangements were made, but even after she had changed reservations at the last moment to come earlier, the baby arrived before she did.

Our friends for the most part expressed interest--the same kind that Martha showed to Judy. "It may be fine for you, but not for me." Then some neighbors were incredulous. One was relieved to find out she'd be away on vacation. Another mother of three didn't think she could stand knowing what was going on across the street.

We weren't looking for confirmation that we had made a correct decision from our friends and neighbors. We felt that we knew what we were doing and we didn't need favorable reactions to assure us of the rightness of our decision. We did need, and received, support from Dr. Brew, the midwife, and, surprisingly, near the end, from a pediatrician--Dr. Herbert Solomon.

AT HOME, WE WOULD BE TOGETHER TO SHARE THE TOTAL EXPERIENCE - THE PLEASANT ASPECTS AS WELL AS THE UNPLEASANT.

AT HOME, RULES FOR INSTITUTIONAL CONVENIENCE AND SAFETY WERE UNNECESSARY.   IF THE BABY WASN'T FOOTPRINTED IMMEDIATELY - OR EVER - HE WAS NOT ABOUT TO BE MIXED UP WITH SOMEONE ELSE'S BABY.

Why was the decision for homebirth so easy when it came? What was in it for us that made it something we really wanted? After discussing these questions with each other we decided that there were four principal needs which constituted the basis for our choice of homebirth: (1) the need for control; (2) responsibility; (3) a private and personal family experience; and (4) familiarity and peacefulness.

Foremost, and underlying our whole enthusiasm for homebirth, was our desire to be in control of the situation. The setting was familiar and comfortable. We could arrange it to suit *our* needs. Instead of us being "intruders" into the medical personnels' world, the midwife and the doctor were visitors. During the process of labor we were freed from having to respond to new and unfamiliar hospital routines and to adjust ourselves to conform to the behavioral expectations of others. Rules for institutional convenience and safety were unnecessary. (If the baby wasn't footprinted immediately - or ever - he was not about to be mixed up with someone else's baby.) At home we were together to share the total experience--pleasant as well as unpleasant aspects.

When we chose prepared childbirth, we accepted certain responsibilities. We learned about the physiological details of labor and delivery and practiced exercises and breathing techniques that we would use to assist the labor and delivery process. We studied the various options for medication and accepted our right to question medical personnel and know what was going on. We wanted to share the experience and take active roles. Deciding to have a homebirth committed us to these responsibilities. Several times we heard from other expectant mothers comments like "Well, if the Lamaze stuff doesn't work, the hospital can take care of me." At home this kind of abdication of responsibility was not possible. Martha's body had to be in good condition. Both of us had to know how to do the breathing and be prepared to carry through on our own. We also needed to provide our own supplies and make arrangements ahead of time with the midwife.

Besides being able to assume responsibility and being in control, we were able, by choosing homebirth, to engender a family-oriented closeness. Older siblings can easily be included in an experience normally denied them, even though the baby will permanently affect their lives. (Some parents prefer not to include older children. But at home, either way the *choice* is theirs to make.) In our case, because the boys are so close in age, our second homebirth prevented the mother-toddler separation trauma. Mommy and Daddy were working at having a baby when Grandma put Derek down for a nap and, as nature would have it, he had a baby brother by the time he woke up.

Not only can homebirth prevent separation of mother and older siblings, it also prevents separation of father, mother, and newborn. Martha could touch our babies immediately. (She actually sat up enough to watch the second one be born. Again, at home, the choice of delivery positions was ours to make.) The mother-infant imprinting took place immediately as the baby opened his eyes and looked into Martha's face. "He's my son." "She's my mother." "Hello." What a wonderful and beautiful moment for all of us to share in our home, in the place where this child was conceived. Bill was able to hold our sons even before they were dressed. Martha nursed them right away. This cements the mother-child bond, stimulates the breasts for quick milk production, and contracts the uterus, helping to prevent postpartum bleeding.

Peacefulness and familiarity were also important to us. For example, when we talked about this, Martha recalled her impressions shortly after delivery. "When everyone went downstairs to eat breakfast the first time, delayed lunch the second, there I was in my own bed with my new son at my breast. My bathroom was right there to be used now or when I wished. Our work was done, for the moment. The result was nestled in my arms. I was at *home* and life continued." There was no "homecoming" to look forward to or to prepare for. We *were* home.

Dr. Solomon, the pediatrician, did not interrupt this feeling when he came to examine our first son, pronouncing him a healthy baby. Unfortunately, he was out of town when our second son arrived and Martha had to take the baby to the doctor's office. It ruined the serenity and closeness engendered in our homebirth atmosphere by jarring mother and son into the outside world rat race via automobile and freeway to make a doctor's appointment on time. The moving out has to happen, but it would have been so much nicer if we could have done it on our own terms as we did with the first baby. Derek's first exposure to the outside world was a trip to church when he was three days old. It was a lovely introduction to the outside world for us as a new family.

Yes, we may be unusual, even peculiar. We needed to be in control of, wanted to assume responsibility for, and chose to participate together in the births of our children. To do this in an atmosphere of familiarity and peacefulness, we chose to have homebirths. Childbirth is a "natural" event for families - something to be enjoyed. We, as responsible, informed adults decided it should happen and be shared in our home.

LEGAL ASPECTS OF HOMEBIRTHS AND OTHER CHILDBIRTH ALTERNATIVES

George J. Annas, JD, MPH*

*Childbirth is not a disease but
a normal function of women.*

Commonwealth v. Porn
196 Mass. 326 (1907)

*Labor and delivery, while a physiologic process,
clearly presents potential hazards to both mother
and fetus before and after birth.   These hazards
require standards of safety which are provided in
the hospital setting and cannot be matched in the
home situation.*

American College of Obstetricians
and Gynecologists   -   May 1975

The law relating to childbirth is complex and varies from
state to state. This account is thus neither exhaustive nor conclusive. Rather, the purpose is to present an overview of the
major issues that courts and legislatures are likely to consider
important when faced with questions involving childbirth in general
and homebirths in particular. The paper is divided into five sections: (1) Changing Hospital Practices in the Courts; (2) Childbirth Assistance, Midwifery, and the Practice of Medicine;
(3) Civil and Criminal Liability Aspects of Homebirths; (4) Some
Questions and Answers; and (5) Summary and Conclusions.

EDITORS' NOTE: The presentation here entitled "Legal Aspects of
Homebirths and Other Childbirth Alternatives" is based on two
sources: (1) "Legal Aspects of Alternative Childbirth Methods,"
a paper by George J. Annas written with the research assistance of
Alice Kupler, JD, copyrighted, 1976, by George J. Annas with permission granted to NAPSAC by George J. Annas to include the paper
in full in this book; and (2) "Legal Aspects of Homebirths," a verbal presentation by George J. Annas given at the NAPSAC Conference,
May, 1976, including a substantial question and answer session.
The article presented here is a combination by the Editors of
these two sources containing the full text of the first copyrighted
paper but modified and amplified throughout with excerpts from the
verbal presentation.

---

    * GEORGE J. ANNAS is Director of the Center for Law and
Health Sciences, Boston University School of Law; Author of "The
Rights of Hospital Patients," Co-Editor of the Book, "Genetics and
the Law," and Editor-in-Chief of the Medicolegal News; he is also
a Member of the Board of Consultants of the International Childbirth
Education Association.

I. Changing Hospital Practices in the Courts

> *If the increasing American trend toward home
> deliveries is to be contained, it is impera-
> tive that an effort be made to make birth in
> the hospital as normal, as homelike, and as
> inexpensive as possible.*

Doris Haire[1]

One method of using the law to encourage changes in hospital
practices is through lawsuits against hospitals, which allege that
the institutions violate the rights of physicians and their patients
by not providing for or permitting the types of services they desire. Courts, however, are extremely reluctant to substitute their
judgement for that of hospital boards of directors. They are thus
likely to continue to defer to their judgements so long as any rational connection with patient safety can be maintained. A review
of the "father-in-the-delivery-room" cases decided to date illus-
trates the strength of judicial preference for "expert" medical
opinion about new procedures and demonstrates that it is unlikely
that desired changes will be mandated by the courts.

While most hospitals with maternity wards currently permit
"husband-coached" childbirth (Lamaze or psychoprophylactic being
the most common method), in which the father is with the mother
throughout labor and delivery, lawsuits to compel a change in the
policies of those institutions that do not allow this procedure
have been universally unsuccessful to date.[2] This is true regardless of whether the hospital is private or public, or whether the
plaintiff is a pregnant woman or her obstetrician.

In the first appellate decision on this question, a Montana
court reversed a lower court ruling in favor of an obstetrician
who had challenged a hospital rule that forbade the presence of
fathers in the delivery room.[3] The administrator of the private,[4]
Catholic hospital contended that the rule was based on a concern
for the spread of infection, chance of an increase in malpractice
suits, possible disturbance of physicians in the doctors' locker
room, increased costs of surgical gowns, potential for invasion of
the privacy of other patients, and was, as well, a measure for the
promotion of staff harmony. Without analyzing the merits of these
contentions, the court concluded simply that as long as minimal
due process was accorded the physician and the rule adopted was
not arbitrary or capricious, the court would not intrude "itself
into the administration of the hospital where the hospital had
acted in good faith on competent medical advice."[5]

The only other case to reach the appellate level in this
area involved a suit by prospective parents against a public hospital.[6] They contended that the hospital's policy denying fathers
a right to be in the delivery room violated the First, Fourth,
Ninth, and Fourteenth Amendments of the United States Constitution,
with specific reference to the "right of marital privacy" enuncia-
ted in the birth control and abortion decisions.

THE LAW WILL NOT FORCE HOSPITALS TO CHANGE WHAT IS ACCEPTED AS "STANDARD MEDICAL PROCEDURE." AS LONG AS THEY SAY THEY HAVE A "REASON" FOR THEIR POLICY, THE COURT IS GOING TO RUBBERSTAMP IT SO THAT HOSPITALS CAN ESSENTIALLY RUN THEIR OWN SHIPS WITH VERY LITTLE THAT CONSUMER GROUPS CAN DO ABOUT IT, WHICH IS OBVIOUSLY ONE REASON PEOPLE GO FOR HOMEBIRTHS.

The lower court dismissed their suit. On appeal the court affirmed the dismissal in a 2:1 decision, with Judge John Paul Stevens writing the majority opinion shortly before his elevation to the United States Supreme Court. In so doing the court made a number of comments which highlight the problems future courts will have to overcome before recognizing a constitutional right of a woman to have the father of her child with her during a hospital delivery.

Perhaps the most important stumbling block is that of precedent. The court was extremely concerned that, were they to find a constitutional right for a husband to be present in the delivery room during childbirth, they would also have to permit "unwed parents" such access. They would "perhaps" be required as well to allow other persons about to undergo serious medical procedures the right to be accompanied by a person of their choice. While I would argue that this might be the most desirable result, I would strongly disagree with the court's view that it is likely to be mandated by a decision of this kind. Childbirth can be distinguished in a number of ways from other procedures - e.g., it is a "natural" process happening to a healthy woman; it is performed in these cases under local or no anesthesia; it is primarily concerned with reproduction; or a combination of these factors (although this would, and certainly *should*, apply to birth by Caesarean section).

It was the court's inability to make such a distinction that reinforced their determination to find against the plaintiffs. In fact, while conceding that "the birth of a child is an event of unequalled importance in the lives of most married couples," the court found the birth procedure itself, "in its medical aspects," to be comparable to other serious hospital procedures," and "extraordinary" in nature! This, of course, rejects the entire rationale of the "natural" childbirth movement, which is that childbirth is normal, not pathological, and that in the vast majority of births little or no medical intervention is either required or desirable.

PARENTS CAN CERTAINLY ASSUME THE RISK OF GIVING BIRTH AT HOME AS CAN INDIVIDUALS WHO HAVE HEART ATTACKS ASSUME THE RISK OF STAYING AT HOME AND TAKING CARE OF THEMSELVES. NO ONE IN THIS SOCIETY HAS TO GO TO THE HOSPITAL FOR ANYTHING - INCLUDING CHILDBIRTH.

The court finally noted that since the plaintiffs only contended that they had a constitutional right if their physician con-
sented to the husband's presence, they had themselves conceded that
good medical practice might at some time require the exclusion of
the husband, and consequently that a hospital might have a rational
basis for finding the procedure unjustified. This, and the recognized "dispute within the medical profession as to the propriety
and safety of permitting the husband to be present during the routine birth," was enough for the court to conclude that it should
not substitute its judgement for that of the hospital board.

The dissenting judge, however, would have reversed the lower
court's ruling and remanded the case for a trial of merits. He
found that the "right of privacy" *did* extend to the delivery room,
and that the evidence before the court (a 1968 survey of ICEA)
demonstrated that of 45,000 cases of fathers in delivery rooms,
"there was not one infection traceable to the practice and not one
malpractice suit." While he conceded that the deprivation of
rights in this case was not of the magnitude of that involved in
the contraception and abortion cases (where access to drugs, de-
vices, and medical services had been forbidden by criminal law),
Judge Sprecher noted that neither was the state's interest of the
same magnitude in this case - an interest which he described as
"so noncompelling as to be virtually nonexistent: The hospital
fears that the participating husband may catch a glimpse of other
women in labor and that it does not have the facilities for him to
don and doff his hospital gown." He concluded by arguing that de-
nial of the mate's presence when the woman desires it "at a critical time is unnecessarily, and I believe unconstitutionally, cruel
to the expectant mother."

THERE IS ONE CHANCE IN 2 MILLION THAT WHEN A PHYSICIAN
SEES A PATIENT THAT THE PATIENT WILL TURN AROUND AND SUE
HIM BECAUSE OF SOMETHING HE DOES. THAT'S EQUIVALENT TO THE
RISK OF DEATH FOR FLYING 100 MILES.

It is worth noting a number of points in this debate. The
first is that courts are likely to continue their tradition of
granting hospital board great latitude in adopting rules or bylaws
that have any rational connection to improved patient care. Moreover, courts will enforce the application of such rules against
individual physicians, patients, or both, provided that the hospital follows some minimal due process requirements (usually set
forth in the hospital's bylaws).[7] Thus, suits challenging hospital rules which prohibit certain procedures, such as Leboyer or
the presence of fathers at birth, are unlikely to be successful.

RED HERRINGS, SUCH AS A POTENTIAL RISE IN MALPRACTICE
SUITS, SHOULD NOT BE PERMITTED TO BLUR THE REAL ISSUES.

Second, red herrings, such as a potential rise in malpractice suits, should not be permitted to blur the real issues. If the courts were convinced that the concealment of malpractice by physicians was the primary reason for denying fathers access to the delivery room, it is highly unlikely that they would sanction such an exclusionary policy. While at least two fathers have sued for emotional trauma suffered by witnessing "the alleged negligent deliveries of their children" (both infants were stillborn),[8] it should be noted that both of these cases were dismissed. The court, after dismissing the cases on a technical ground, noted that the cases would probably have failed on the independent ground that the fathers were *voluntary* witnesses to the tragedy, and thus assumed the potential risk of such a happening. The principal allegation, however, was negligence in the delivery and the suits would probably have been filed whether or not the father had been present.

THERE ARE ABOUT A DOZEN CASES SO FAR WHERE PEOPLE HAVE GONE TO COURT TO TRY TO GET HOSPITALS TO CHANGE THEIR POLICIES TO PERMIT HUSBANDS TO ACCOMPANY THEIR WIVES IN LABOR AND DELIVERY. ALL OF THESE CASES HAVE BEEN UNSUCCESSFUL. IT DOESN'T MATTER WHETHER IT'S A PUBLIC HOSPITAL, A PRIVATE HOSPITAL, WHETHER THE PARENTS SUE, OR THE DOCTOR SUES - ALL HAVE BEEN UNSUCCESSFUL.

Finally, it should be apparent from this discussion that the courts are *not* the forum in which the *real* issues at stake are likely to be addressed. Those issues involve the desire of many couples to have a more human, joyful, and family-centered experience during childbirth than is possible at many technologically oriented hospitals. It is a consumer rebellion against the medical model indiscriminantly applied to all pregnant women that is the heart of this debate. While minor victories in this battle may be won in the courts, civil litigation is not a terribly effective method of promoting safe alternatives to present childbirth methods. The proper arenas are likely to be the state legislatures and health regulatory agencies, and the proper issue is consumer influence on the way childbirth services are delivered.

NO TWO LAWYERS WOULD GIVE YOU THE SAME IDEA OF WHAT THE LAW IS ABOUT ON HOMEBIRTH BECAUSE, FOR ONE THING, THERE IS VERY LITTLE LAW DIRECTLY ON HOMEBIRTH. IN FACT, ALL OF THE CONCLUSIONS GIVEN HERE HAD TO BE DRAWN BY ANALOGY FROM LESS THAN 2 DOZEN CASES OVER THE LAST 200 YEARS, IF YOU CAN BELIEVE THAT, AND FROM JUST A HANDFUL OF STATUTES FROM A NUMBER OF STATES, ALMOST ALL OF THEM ON MIDWIFERY.

II. Childbirth Assistance, Midwifery, and the Practice of Medicine

> *Today, though independent midwifery is illegal*
> *in parts of the United States, it continues to·*
> *be practiced and respected throughout the rest*
> *of the world.*

Suzanne Arms[9]

The area of the law that has been most active in the field of childbirth is that related to midwifery. Developments have occurred in both the courts and the state legislatures, and both are worth reviewing.

A. The Courts

In the courts the legal issue generally presented is whether or not the practice of midwifery, involving assistance at a home-birth, is the practice of medicine (in which case only a physician may engage in the activity without violating the criminal law). The leading case on this subject arose in 1907 in Massachusetts.[10] In that case, a woman admitted to having delivered "many women in childbirth for compensation," having sometimes used "obstetrical instruments" in emergencies (but never if a physician could be called in time), and using "six printed prescriptions or formulas" in treating her patients. These latter were to be used "For vaginal douche," "For post-partum hemorrhage," "To prevent purulent ophthalmia in the new-born." "For after-pains," "For uterine inertia," and "For painful hemorrhoids or piles." She was a trained and experienced nurse and a graduate of the Chicago Midwife Institute.

The sole question before the Massachusetts Supreme Judicial Court was whether or not this activity constituted the practice of medicine. The court concluded that "although childbirth is not a disease, but a normal function of women" the practice of medicine is not confined solely to diseases, and obstetrics is commonly recognized as an "important branch of the science of medicine." The court noted further that the treatment of the infant's eyes was, in any event, not a duty of a midwife, and accordingly a jury could lawfully find that the defendant, Hanna Porn, was engaged in the practice of medicine. This conclusion, the court said, was mandated by the state's practice of medicine statute, and would have been different had the state legislature passed a statute that distinguished the practice of midwifery from the practice of medicine.

The next significant case to be decided arose in Texas in 1956. The defendant, Omar Blake Rowland, was charged with unlawfully treating a pregnant woman for an agreed-upon fee of $40.00.[11] The evidence showed that midwifery had been the defendant's occupation since 1924 and that she had delivered thousands of babies in the Houston area. The issue before the Texas Court of Criminal Appeals was whether or not to overturn her misdemeanor conviction for practicing medicine unlawfully. The court cited the Porn case described above as the only case on point. However, the court

found that "the legislature of Texas has not defined the practice
of medicine so as to include the act of assisting women in parturition or childbirth . . ."

The Texas court found further that a number of other statutes
indicated that such practice was lawful. These included a statute
requiring "all doctors, midwives, nurses, or those in attendance
at childbirth to use prophylactic drops in the child's eyes," a
statute regarding the reporting of stillbirths that said in part,
that "Midwives shall not sign certificates of stillbirths" if a
physician is not in attendance at the birth, and a statute authorizing midwives to sign birth certificates. From these considera-
tions the court concluded that the practice of midwifery by a non-
licensed individual could not be considered a violation of Texas
law and accordingly reversed her conviction.

> THE LAW IS OUTCOME ORIENTED. UNLESS SOMETHING GOES
> WRONG, THE LAW IS NOT LIKELY TO AFFECT ANYTHING THAT
> PEOPLE DO IN OUR SOCIETY.

The most recent case involving this issue is in California
where a state and municipal court held that midwifery *was* the
practice of medicine but were overruled in early 1976 by the California Superior Court which held that midwifery *was not* necessarily the practice of medicine.[12] Now, in May, 1976, the Superior
Court has reversed itself so that the issue is back on appeal
again. The law in California is probably one of the most confused
of any state, but the main point is that the law varies from state
to state, so when it comes to the law, you have to know the law of
your state.

The foregoing case arose after the arrest of a number of the
individuals working at the Santa Cruz Birth Center. The arrests
occurred after a pregnant woman employee in the California State
Department of Consumer Affairs approached the Birth Center for help
in a homebirth. About a month before she was due to deliver she
called the Center, stating that she was in labor. Two women from
the Center came to her home where a number of men, dressed as hippies, stated that the pregnant woman was in the shower, asked if
they were midwives, gave them $50, identified themselves as under-
cover agents, and arrested them. Simultaneously a raid was carried
out at the Birth Center and most of their files and equipment were
confiscated.[13]

The defendants asked the Superior Court to issue an injunc-
tion restraining the municipal court and the state from proceeding
with the prosecution on the grounds that the statute regarding
practicing medicine without a license was unconstitutionally vague
and that assisting at homebirths was not a violation of the statute.
The court refused. On appeal, the higher court found the statute
was constitutional, but found also that it prohibited only treatment of "any ailment, blemish, deformity, disease, disfigurement,

disorder, injury, or other mental or physical condition of any person . . ." The court determined that the phrase, "other mental or
physical condition," referred to conditions like those specifically
enumerated, and accordingly that "undertaking to assist and treat a
woman in pregnancy and childbirth" was not an offense under the
statute, since "pregnancy and childbirth are not diseases but rather are normal physiological functions of women." The court
therefore ruled that the charges against the Birth Center defendants must be dismissed.[14] This ruling in favor of the Santa Cruz
midwives was in early 1976 but now, in May, 1976, as was stated
earlier, the court has reversed itself so that the issue in California continues to be a matter of debate.

The major conclusion from these cases is, of course, that
defining what is or is not the practice of medicine is a matter for
the state legislatures, and they may rule on this matter as they
see fit. Therefore, the state legislatures are the most appropriate arena to work for change in states where change is desired.

B. The Legislatures

Approximately forty states have statutes dealing with the
practice of midwifery, and many of these statutes have undergone
significant revision within the past five years.[15] Before such revisions the typical midwife statute read similarly to the one now in
force in Minnesota:

> A person desiring to practice midwifery in the
> state, if not already licensed to do so, should
> apply to the state Board of Medical Examiners
> for a license. The license should be granted
> upon the production of a diploma from a school
> of midwifery recognized by the Board, or after
> examination upon the consent of seven members
> thereof.[16]

The modern trend (so far adopted by about ten states) is to
adopt a statute similar to that now in effect in Ohio. It requires
that one must hold a diploma from a college for nurse midwives,
pass an examination, be of good moral character, and hold a degree
in nursing. Licensed nurse midwives may only work under the direct
supervision of a physician and may not deal with any complicated
births, use any instruments, or treat any abnormal condition except
in an emergency.[17] The position of both the American College of
Obstetricians & Gynecologists and the American College of Nurse-Midwives
is that nurse midwives should only assist in hospital-based deliveries, and that homebirths should be discouraged. These statutes,
of course, support this position. The legislative trend is, thus,
to make it illegal for licensed nurse midwives to attend homebirths
(unless accompanied by a physician).

THE POSITION OF BOTH THE ACOG AND THE ACNM IS THAT NURSE
MIDWIVES SHOULD ONLY ASSIST IN HOSPITAL-BASED DELIVERIES
AND THAT HOMEBIRTHS SHOULD BE DISCOURAGED.

THE TOPIC, "WHAT IS THE LAW ABOUT HOMEBIRTHS?" IS LIKE A FINAL EXAM QUESTION IN LAW SCHOOL WHERE THEY GIVE YOU A FACT SITUATION AND SAY, "TELL US WHO CAN SUE WHO FOR WHAT." AND THE ANSWER IS "ALMOST ANYONE CAN SUE ALMOST EVERYONE FOR ALMOST EVERY-THING." BUT THE RELEVANT QUESTIONS ARE, "HOW LIKELY IS IT THAT ANYBODY IS GOING TO SUE YOU?" AND IF SOMEONE DOES, "WHAT'S THE RISK THAT YOU ARE GOING TO LOSE?"

III. Civil and Criminal Liability Aspects of Homebirths

> We talked about risk. I knew that I or the
> baby could die. We decided the benefits of
> homebirth were worth the risk. When my baby
> was born, she lay in a kind of primordial
> state before she cried.   I thought she was
> dead and I accepted it.   She cried then.

Unidentified mother[18]

The law is generally concerned with outcomes. Therefore, except in the case of the unlawful practice of medicine or mid-wifery (discussed above), or unless the mother or child dies or is permanently disabled in the process of childbirth at home, it is unlikely that there would or could be any legal action taken against the parents, a friend of the family, a midwife, or a phy-sician for participating in a homebirth. Moreover, the mother will probably be found to have knowledgeably assumed the risk of homebirth in regard to herself, and therefore be barred from suing anyone for her own injury or death in the absence of negligence. Thus, legal liability in the absence of negligence is likely to be significant only in the case where the infant dies or is seriously and permanently disabled because the birth took place at home. This discussion will, accordingly, concentrate on the case where the child dies after birth at home and where it could be demon-strated that the child would have lived had it been delivered in a hospital. If this latter point cannot be demonstrated, no cri-minal or civil action based on the child's death is likely to be successful.

A. The Parents

All the case law that exists directly on point indicates that neither parent will be legally liable for failure to obtain medical care or assistance *prior* to the birth of the child.   In 1860, for example, a British judge refused to submit a manslaughter charge to the jury in the case of a woman who failed to seek medi-cal assistance during labor.[19] In 1904 another British trial judge ruled that a mother's duty to provide medical care for her child commenced only *after* birth.[20] Relying on these two cases, the Wyoming Supreme Court in 1954 reversed the manslaughter con-viction of a mother whose infant died shortly after birth.[21]

The court noted that it could find no legal authority for imposing a duty on a woman about to give birth to seek medical assistance, and accordingly affirmed the rule that an infant must be born before the parents' duty of care commences. One legal commentator has, however, suggested that the before-after birth dichotomy cannot withstand critical scrutiny and has argued that "where circumstances make the possible need for medical care clear, failure to obtain care that leads to the infant's death should be culpable."[22] This probably is the better rule, and one that the courts might well apply in cases where the mother had reason to know that hers was a "high risk" pregnancy where a hospital birth was strongly indicated.

THERE IS NO CRIMINAL LIABILITY FOR STILLBIRTHS. IF THE BABY DIES SHORTLY AFTER BIRTH AT HOME, THERE IS THE POSSIBILITY OF A CHARGE OF MANSLAUGHTER IF IMMEDIATE MEDICAL CARE HAD NOT BEEN SOUGHT. BUT NO PHYSICIAN, NO NURSE MIDWIFE, NO PARENT, NO ONE HAS EVER BEEN BROUGHT UP ON A MANSLAUGHTER CHARGE FOR THIS IF EFFORTS WERE MADE TO SUMMON APPROPRIATE MEDICAL CARE.

Under either approach, however, it is clear that once the child is born the parents do have a legal obligation to provide it with indicated medical care, and failure to do so constitutes child neglect that could support a homicide conviction.[23] While the liability of the mother immediately after birth for failure to take care of the infant is not likely to be great (in the absence of prior knowledge that trouble should have been anticipated),[24] the father could be held for any failure to summon or seek the needed medical assistance for the child.

In one 1905 case, for example, the judge instructed the jury that a father could be found liable for manslaughter in the death of his infant for neglecting his duty "when the woman was in the pains and perils of childbirth" to summon aid.[25] In a similar case, the Kentucky Supreme Court decided that no homicide conviction could stand against a husband who failed to summon medical care for his wife during childbirth when the failure was due to his wife's insistence.[26] In a case in which the wife died, the husband began assisting in the delivery but became alarmed about his wife's condition, and summoned medical aid. The court found the wife to have been well-educated and desirous of having her baby at home.

All of these cases illustrate that when a death occurs during a homebirth the state may feel that a wrong has been committed against society and accordingly prosecute for negligent homicide. This result may be even more likely in the 1970's than these early cases indicate since the custom of having children in hospitals is certainly more widespread and accepted now than it was at the time these cases were decided, and the standard an individual will be measured against is what a reasonably prudent person in the community would do under like circumstances at the present time.

B. The Birth Attendant

Licensed midwives, operating under the authority of state
statute, will be held criminally liable only in cases of extreme
gross negligence or wilful and wanton conduct, and will be held
civilly liable only if they fail to perform up to the standards of
their profession. A licensed physician might be held criminally
liable under similar circumstances, and civilly liable for malpractice if he is negligent in the delivery if he failed to perform up
to the standards of his profession. An argument can be made, although it is unlikely to be successful, that in some communities
the standard of medical care is that all births must be in hospitals, and therefore it is negligence *per se* for a physician to
attend a homebirth. This approach should be rejected on policy
grounds, in that it would not deter those persons who are committed
to having their children at home from doing so, but only make it
impossible for them to obtain medical assistance if they desired
it. Moreover, in the matter of childbirth it is possible that,
following the reasoning used in the United States Supreme Court's
abortion decisions, a physician could be found to have a constitutional right to practice medicine as he and his patient see fit,
subject to review only by the Board of Registration of Medicine
in his state.[27]

TO WIN A NEGLIGENCE SUIT FOR HAVING A HOMEBIRTH, THE
PEOPLE HAVE TO PROVE THAT EITHER THE MOTHER OR THE CHILD
WAS PERMANENTLY DAMAGED AND THAT IF THEY HAD BEEN IN THE HOSPITAL
THEY WOULD NOT HAVE BEEN DAMAGED. IF YOU CAN PROVE THAT WHATEVER
HAPPENED WOULD HAVE HAPPENED NO MATTER WHERE YOU WERE, NOBODY CAN
SUE YOU FOR ANYTHING.

On the other hand, a physician will not be found liable for
abandonment in a case where the physician indicates that he will
not perform a home delivery and later refuses to render assistance
when his patient calls him during childbirth. In one case, for
example, the physician told his patient that the only proper place
for a delivery was in the hospital "where proper facilities were
available" and refused to attend her at home. She hired a midwife
but complications developed during the delivery and the physician,
and two others, were called. All refused to attend and the child
died. The court refused to hold that the defendant physician was
negligent for not responding to her call for help.[28]

YOU CAN ALWAYS REFUSE A MEDICAL PROCEDURE; BUT YOU CANNOT
DICTATE MEDICAL PROCEDURE. YOU DO NOT HAVE TO ACCEPT WHAT
A DOCTOR OFFERS, BUT NEITHER CAN YOU TELL HIM WHAT TO DO.

IV. Some Questions and Answers (see Editors' Note on p. 176)

Q. WHAT IS THE LEGAL LIABILITY OF INDIVIDUALS (NOT PROFESSIONALS) INVOLVED IN A HOMEBIRTH?

A. The law is such that unless something serious goes wrong, there would be no legal liability. Now when I say "serious" I mean something like the child being permanently disabled or the child or mother dying. If a complication ensues and you have to be hospitalized and it is corrected, then this is not a problem. There has to be death or a permanent disability. And if that happens, what are the possibilities? There are two legal things that could happen: There could be a civil suit where somebody sues you for money damages. The other thing that could happen is a criminal suit where somebody wants to put you in jail or fine you.

Q. WHO'S LIABLE IF A MOTHER DIES IN A MEDICALLY UNATTENDED HOMEBIRTH?

A. If the mother dies I don't think there is any legal liability for anybody as long as the mother knew what she was doing. There have not been any cases where courts have ruled that the mother has an obligation to seek medical assistance in childbirth. Mothers can assume the risk of giving birth at home as can individuals who have heart attacks assume the risk of staying at home and taking care of themselves or having their families taking care of them. No one is this society has to go to the hospital for anything - including childbirth.

Q. WHAT IS THE PARENTS' LEGAL OBLIGATION TO THE CHILD IN AN UNATTENDED HOMEBIRTH?

A. As of 1963, all 50 states in the U.S. passed laws dealing with child abuse and child neglect. These are really the critical laws to look at in homebirths. Is what you're doing child abuse? If it is not child abuse or child neglect, then there is really no legal problem. The case law says that you can't abuse your fetus. Some states are changing this to make laws against feticide, for example, which is killing the fetus in the third trimester. But this really has very little to do with homebirth. The law now is that you have no obligation to your child, no legal obligation until it is born--i.e. from the moment it is expelled from the mother. From then on, if the child is in need of medical assistance, you have the obligation to provide it with that assistance. If it has to go to the hospital and you failed to make every effort to get there and the baby dies, that's manslaughter. Under certain circumstances an ambitious district attorney could even bring a charge of first-degree murder since he could say that you had the birth at home intentionally and after it was born you intentionally did not give it needed medical attention. But I wouldn't expect that to ever happen. I would expect that people having homebirths would make every effort to get to the hospital if the baby needed it. Now, if the infant does not need medical care, and most don't obviously, there is no problem if medical advice is not sought.

Q. HOW LIKELY IS A MANSLAUGHTER CHARGE IN THE CASE OF THE BABY
DYING?

A. I think this is the main criminal possibility, but as a
matter of fact, no one has ever been brought up on a manslaughter charge for this in a typical homebirth situation. No physician, no nurse midwife, no parent. I don't say it never
happened because it did in 1907, but it hasn't happened in
recent history and in that case the woman died. Since she was
well educated and knew what she was doing, the husband could
not be held responsible. So it seems to me that criminal
liability, though possible, is not very likely, even if the
child dies, because it seems to me that people having homebirths
would take their kids to the hospital if they needed to and
if they do that, there is no liability. For stillbirths,
there is no criminal liability.

Q. WHAT IS THE POSSIBILITY OF CIVIL LIABILITY IN HOMEBIRTH?

A. You can always be sued as parents or as a birth attendant
for negligence if you do something that someone in your position would not do. If you are a physician or a midwife, you
would have to live up to the standard of your respective profession. If you are negligent, you can always be sued.

Q. WHAT IF YOU ARE NOT NEGLIGENT BUT SOMETHING GOES WRONG ANYWAY,
CAN YOU BE SUED THEN?

A. The first thing to determine is whether it would have gone
wrong in the hospital or did it go wrong because you were at
home. To win a negligence suit, people have to prove that
there was damage to the mother or the child and that if you had
been in the hospital the damage would not have happened. If
you can prove that whatever happened would have happened no
matter where you were, nobody can sue you for anything and
expect to win. But now you have to realize that anybody can
sue you for anything--the question is are they going to win.

Q. WHAT ABOUT THE CHILD SUING ITS PARENTS?

A. If he did, what he would allege is that his parents were
negligent in having a homebirth. Before he can have grounds to
do that there must be some permanent disability that can be
proven to have been caused by not being in the hospital and
which would not have happened had the birth been in the hospital. In most states, the child can sue his parents up to the
age of 21--three years after he reaches the age of majority.
But what's the likelihood of that happening? What is the likelihood of a child suing his parents because he is retarded?
Or for some other problem? You can answer that as well as I.
I don't know of any such cases ever happening like that. It
is a possibility, but certainly a remote one.

Q.   ARE THE LIABILITIES FOR DOCTORS THE SAME AS FOR MIDWIVES?

A.   No. The professions have different standards and as long
as the physician, the lay midwife, or the nurse midwife lives
up to the standards of their respective professions I can see
almost no possibility of making any legal headway against them.
There is a greater problem with physicians because it is
possible that a court or jury might find that the standard
medical practice is to have a child in the hospital and that
the doctor was negligent, per se. The attitude would be that
no physician of standing in the profession would attend a
homebirth and therefore, the physician should absolutely be
liable for anything that goes on. Now, that has never happened
before but it could. Physicians are at a much higher risk than
are lay midwives or nurse midwives because they are held to a
much higher standard of care. Now you and I and all the midwives may know that the physician probably knows less about
normal childbirth than the average midwife, but the court and
the jury are going to think that he knows a lot more and that
he should have known better.

Q.   HOW GREAT IS THE THREAT OF MALPRACTICE SUITS TO PHYSICIANS?

A.   Physicians say that there is a malpractice crisis in the
United States. They say that they are being sued no matter
what they do and that they don't want to do things because of
the risk of suing.   Well, the risk of a physician being sued
for malpractice, for anything now, for each doctor-patient
contact, is approximately 1 in 2 million. I mean there is
only one chance in 2 million of a physician who sees an individual patient that that patient will turn around and sue him
for something he does. That is equivalent, if you like
equivalent risks, to death for flying 100 miles. I think
that is almost trivial. You don't even think about the risk
of flying 100 miles. You fly 500 miles and its five times the
risk of being sued for malpractice. Now by comparison, the
risk of death from general anesthesia is 1 in 6,000. It is
obviously a much more serious risk because not only is one
more likely but one is for loss of money while the other is for
life. Yet, physicians will tell you that they don't feel it
necessary to mention this to their patients because it is a
"trivial" risk. "It is not statistically significant," they
say. And yet they are concerned about something on the order
of one chance in a million for malpractice.

Q.   CAN PARENTS SIGN A WAIVER OF MEDICAL NEGLIGENCE FOR A MIDWIFE
OR DOCTOR ATTENDING A HOMEBIRTH?

A.   You can't waive negligence. People, doctors, midwives, all
have to live up to some standards. They can't say, "Okay I
will only attend you if you'll hold me harmless for negligence,
like if I forget to cut the umbilical cord or if you hemorrhage
or something." I mean, that would be crazy. You don't want to
do that. The real question is can they hold you harmless if

something happens regardless of negligence, something that you
didn't cause to happen. And yes, they can. It seems to me
they can, as long as they are fully informed. As long as they
know what the risks are, then they can say, "Yes, I'll assume
the risks of a homebirth," but that doesn't include the risk
of being negligent like dropping the baby, etc.

Q. SHOULD BIRTH ATTENDANTS OBTAIN A SIGNED AND WRITTEN STATEMENT
OF INFORMED CONSENT FROM PARENTS?

A. I recommend it mainly just as a check on yourself to make
sure that you have told the patient everything you think they
should know. And in the rare event you get sued, it is protection for yourself too. But I like written informed consents
mainly as a check on people's memories so that everybody knows
what the significant risks are and everybody has a copy of it,
so there's no misunderstanding. People usually forget oral
consent.

Q. DOES THE AMERICAN MEDICAL ASSOCIATION HAVE AN ANTI-HOMEBIRTH
POLICY?

A. I don't know about the AMA. But the American College of
Obstetricians and Gynecologists and the American College of
Nurse Midwives do not give official sanction to any out-of-
hospital alternative.

Q. CAN A HOSPITAL THREATEN A PRIVATE GROUP PRACTICE WITH LEGAL
ACTION IF THE PRIVATE GROUP ENGAGES IN HOMEBIRTHS?

A. Anybody can threaten you for almost anything as long as it
doesn't become an assault. They can also take away your hospital privileges and then you can sue on the grounds that the
hospital by law forbidding participation in homebirths is
wrong. Then you are into the courts and we have already seen
that they are conservative. Is the court going to say, "the
hospital is wrong and homebirth is good." Or are they going
to say "standard medical procedure says homebirths are bad."
Even if the homebirth issue is not mentioned in the hospital
bylaws, the courts would probably support the hospital.

Q. CAN A DOCTOR GO OVER HOSPITAL POLICIES IN ALLOWING HUSBANDS TO
BE PRESENT AT BIRTH?

A. It depends on the hospital. But in some hospitals the
doctor can have whoever he wants there. Obviously he can bring
medical students or residents or interns and never ask you for
permission. They can bring in husbands if they want to. In
general, you can do almost anything on a "one shot" basis. It
is when you try to change the policy for everyone that hospitals
get upset.

Q. WHAT CAN A HOSPITAL DO IF THE FATHER JUST WALKS INTO THE DELI-
VERY ROOM?

A. The hospital could probably try to use physical force if
it wanted to, but that would probably be more trouble than it
was worth. That could involve an assault. I don't think it
is necessarily a trespass on the part of the husband to want
to stay with his wife. It is my own view that the hospital
could legally call the sheriff and ask him to remove the husband
as a trespasser. It is about the only thing they could do
besides just getting upset at you or sending the head nurse
to talk down to you and try to get you to leave. In return
you could threaten to call your lawyer or the newspaper. In
general, as long as it is a one shot deal, hospitals don't
do anything. As long as you can threaten to make more trouble
for them than it's worth, they will just say, "Well you are
just crazy" and they will tell everybody and start excusing
you. They'll say, "Well, you are going to have to be careful
in that room because she's a little crazy." But if you are
willing to go through that, it is not a problem. You can almost
get anything you want in the hospital by doing that. It is
cheaper than suing.

Q. HOW ABOUT THE SILVER NITRATE IN A HOMEBIRTH? WHAT CAN THEY DO
IF YOU DON'T USE IT?

A. It depends on the state and states vary widely. In Massachusetts putting silver nitrate in the baby's eyes is considered
practicing medicine so that if you are not a physician it is
actually illegal to do it. In Texas anyone who is present at
the birth is legally obliged to give silver nitrate--whether
he is a midwife, a physician, or whatever.

Q. CAN WE REFUSE A MEDICAL PROCEDURE?

A. Yes. You can refuse any medical procedure. But you can't
dictate medical procedure. You can't tell professionals how to
do procedures on you. You can refuse any procedure, including
silver nitrate. You can refuse any treatment, but you can't
demand certain kinds of treatment. You can't tell a doctor how
to deliver a child. You can refuse X, Y, and Z position. You
can refuse any drugs. You can refuse an episiotomy. But you
can't tell them to do this or that.

EDITORS' NOTE: The foregoing questions and answers were gleaned
from the taped transcript of the NAPSAC Conference and were given
extemporaneously by Dr. Annas. Between that and the necessary
paraphrasing there are doubtless some technical errors. For
clarification on any of these points, please write Dr. Annas,
address given on p. 182 of this book. If your question concerns
laws in your own state, it would be best to consult a lawyer in
your state.

V. Summary and Conclusions

Three main points have been made here: (1) the law is very conservative and is likely to reflect the established standard medical practice; (2) the law varies from state to state; and (3) the law is outcome oriented--unless something goes wrong the law is not likely to affect us.

In general, the law concerning childbirth is archaic and supports the conservative nature of "standard medical practice." This is illustrated by Judge John Paul Stevens' opinion that "in its medical aspects, the obstetrical procedure is comparable to other serious hospital procedures . . ."[16] No court that has considered the question has required hospitals to change their procedures to permit fathers in the delivery room or any other safe "alternative" childbirth method desired by the physician and the pregnant woman.

This approach, however, is a classic two-edged sword. In classifying childbirth as a "serious hospital procedure," courts insure that the patient about to give birth is protected fully by the doctrine of informed consent. This doctrine requires the physician to fully inform the patient as to the risks (e.g., of anesthesia to both mother and child), alternatives (e.g., regarding positioning and drugs used), and major problems of recuperation of both mother and child involved in each alternative.[29] Such information should, of course, be conveyed well before the date of delivery, the woman and her physician should discuss the issues, and an agreement should be reached.

The law on midwives is undergoing signigicant changes in many states. The current trend is to require more training and formal certification for midwives, and to require that they work under the supervision of a physician. This latter requirement generally limits them to assisting at hospital births only.

The law may also inhibit both parents and physicians from utilizing the alternative of homebirth. The law on such births is mostly to be found in lower court opinions from the early part of this century. Most seem to assume that a hospital-based, or at least a doctor-attended, birth is the only "acceptable" medical choice. The law is, however, primarily concerned with results, and no civil or criminal action is likely against parents or midwives who participate in a homebirth in which no harm comes to mother or child. In the rare case, however, where the child is injured - and one can demonstrate that if the birth had taken place in a hospital the injury would have been avoided - criminal actions for child abuse (or manslaughter if the child dies) are possible, as a future civil suit by the child against any person assisting at the birth. Should a physician assist at a homebirth and the child be similarly injured, the child might likewise bring a malpractice action against the physician if he or she can show (as they currently could) that "good medical practice" mandated a hospital-based delivery.

There are many cases where surviving husbands have recovered substantial verdicts following the death of their wives because of improperly administered anesthetics during childbirth, and the number of lawsuits involving permanent injury to mothers and babies in hospital-based deliveries is proliferating. Nevertheless, most judges and legislators probably believe that a hospital delivery is less dangerous than a home delivery - even though the opposite may be true with the normal delivery.

Civil litigation, as illustrated by the fathers in the delivery room cases, is not a terribly effective method of promoting safe alternatives to present childbirth methods. What is needed is a change in the definition of "good medical practice" that courts will accept. Two approaches are possible. One is to pass state statutes defining the circumstances under which homebirths or other alternatives are acceptable medical practice (or to have the state medical licensing board promulgate regulations defining this). The other is the far more difficult task of getting the medical profession, especially the obstetricians, to change its practices to conform to patient desires in a manner consistent with the health of both mother and child.

MOST JUDGES AND LEGISLATORS PROBABLY BELIEVE THAT A HOSPITAL DELIVERY IS LESS DANGEROUS THAN A HOME DELIVERY, EVEN THOUGH THE OPPOSITE MAY BE TRUE WITH THE NORMAL DELIVERY.

REFERENCES

1. D. Haire, The Cultural Warping of Childbirth, ICEA, 1972 at 16.

2. As a result of a notice in the Fall, 1975, issue of the Newsletter of the International Childbirth Education Association, printed courtesy of the ICEA President, Peg Beals, RN, I have been informed of cases in St. Cloud, Minnesota, St. Joseph, Missouri, Fort Myers, Florida, & Baton Rouge, Louisiana, Owensboro, Kentucky, and Valparaiso, Indiana, none of which has been successful to date.

3. St. Vincent's Hospital v. Hulit, 520 p.2d 99 (Mont. 1974).

4. On the issue of whether there is a right to judicial review of a private hospital's decision-making process, the court said: "We need not here decide that issue, but will assume that such a review is proper."

5. It is of interest to note that while the court lifted the temporary restraining order, the hospital has apparently continued to permit fathers in the delivery room. (Private communication, Peg Beals, Nov. 11, 1975).

REFERENCES CONT'D

6. Fitzgerald v. Porter Memorial Hospital, 523 F.2d 716 (7th Cir. 1975).

7. See Fahey v. Holy Family Hospital, 336 N.E. 2d 309 (Ill. 1975); Khan v. Suburban Comm. Hospital, 340 N.E. 2d 398 (Ohio 1976); Sosa v. Bd. of Managers of Val Verde Mem. Hospital, 437 F.2d 173 (5th Cir. 1971).

8. Justus v. Atchison, Powell v. Atchison, 126 Cal Rptr. 150 (Ct. App. 2d Dist. 1975).

9. S. Arms, Immaculate Deception, Houghton-Mifflin, Boston, 1975 at 151.

10. Commonwealth v. Porn, 196 Mass. 326 (1907).

11. Banti v. State, 289 S.W. 2d 244 (Tex. Ct. Crim. App. 1956).

12. Bowland v. Municipal Court, 54 C.A. 3d 810 (Cal. Ct. App. 1st Dist. 1976).

13. As told in S. Arms, Immaculate Deception, Houghton-Mifflin Co., Boston, 1975, at 210-219.

14. Effective Sept. 23, 1974, California's laws were amended by adding a section on "Midwifery" providing for a certificate to practice midwifery, authorizing the holder to attend and assist a woman in normal childbirth, and prescribing what a midwife may or may not do. This statute was in no way involved in the Bowland opinion.

15. A special issue of the Journal of Nurse Midwifery, scheduled to be published in the summer of 1976, will catalog and explain state statutes and regulations on midwifery. I am grateful to Elizabeth M. Cooper, CNM, Coordinator of the Legislative Information System of the American College of Nurse Midwives Legislation Committee for a summary of this information.

16. Minn. St. Anno. sec. 148.31.

17. Ohio St. sec. 4731.30-4731.34.

18. Mother quoted in M. Edwards, Unattended Homebirths, 73 Am. J. Nursing 1332, Aug. 1973.

19. Regina v. Knights, 175 Eng. Rep. 952 (1860).

20. Rex v. Izod, 20 Cox Crim. Cas. 690 (Oxford Cir. 1904).

21. State v. Osmus, 73 Wyo. 183, 276 P.2d 469 (1954).

22. J. Robertson, Involuntary Euthanasia of Defective Newborns:
A Legal Analysis, 27 Stanford L. Rev. 213, 218 fn. 34, citing
State v. Shepherd, 255 Iowa 1218, 124 N.W. 2d 712 (1963).

23. Id. at 218-230.

24. Although in at least one case a mother has been found
guilty of manslaughter in the death of her infant where she
delivered her illegitimate child alone and unattended in her
bathroom. She failed to tie the umbilical cord and the baby
died shortly after birth from hemorrhaging. People v. Chavez, 176
p.2d 92 (Cal. 1947).

25. Commonwealth v. Signerski, 14 Pa. Dist. 361 (1905)

26. Westrup V. Commonwealth, 123 Ky. 95, 93 S.W. 646 (1906).

27. "If a physician is licensed by the State, he is recognized
by the State as capable of exercising acceptable clinical judgement. If he fails in this, professional censure or deprivation
of his license are available remedies. Required acquiescence by
co-practitioners has no rational connection with a patient's
needs and unduly infringes on the physician's right to practice."
Doe v. Bolton, 93 S. Ct. 739, 751 (1973).

28. Vindrine v. Mayes, 127 So. 2d 809 (Ct. App. La. 1961).

29. Annas, GJ: The Rights of Hospital Patients, Avon Books,
New York, 1975.

Addresses of Authors

George J. Annas, JD, MPH
Center for Law & Health Sciences
Boston University School of Law
209 Bay State Road
Boston, Massachusetts 02215

James D. Brew, MD
Yater Clinic
1780 Massachusetts Avenue NW
Washington, DC 20036

Hart Collins
Neil Collins, JD
2704 Barmettler Street
Raleigh, North Carolina 27607

Ludovic J. DeVocht, MD
4421 Seminary Road
Alexandria, Virginia 22304

Mayer Eisenstein, MD
664 North Michigan Avenue
Suite 600
Chicago, Illinois 60611

Janet L. Epstein, RN, CNM
Maternity Center Associates, Ltd.
5415 Cedar Lane, Suite 107-B
Bethesda, Maryland 20014

Frederic Ettner, MD
2118 Maple Avenue
Evanston, Illinois 60201

Doris Haire, DMS
American Foundation for Maternal
    and Child Health
30 Beekman Place
New York, New York 10022

Betty Hosford, RN, CNM
401 Central Avenue
Cranford, New Jersey 07016

Cedar Koons
Stephen Koons
1014 Burch Avenue
Durham, NC 27705

Martha Longbrake, RN
William Longbrake, DBA
5901 Bryn Mawr Road
College Park, Maryland 20740

Ruth Watson Lubic, RN, CNM
Maternity Center Association
48 East 92nd Street
New York, New York 10028

Marion F. McCartney, RN, CNM
Maternity Center Associates, Ltd.
5415 Cedar Lane, Suite 107-B
Bethesda, Maryland 20014

Lewis E. Mehl, MD
Inst. for Childbirth & Fam. Res.
2522 Dana Street
Berkeley, CA 94704

Robert S. Mendelsohn, MD
664 North Michigan Avenue
Suite 600
Chicago, Illinois 60611

Nancy Mills
7351 Covey Road
Forestville, California 95436

Lee Stewart, CCE
David Stewart, PHD
Rt. 1, Box 300
Marble Hill, MO 63764

Marian Tompson
La Leche League International
9616 Minneapolis Avenue
Franklin Park, Illinois 60131

FOR QUESTIONS PERTAINING TO ANY OF THE ARTICLES PUBLISHED
HEREIN, PLEASE WRITE DIRECTLY TO THE AUTHORS THEMSELVES.

AMERICAN COLLEGE OF HOME OBSTETRICS

2821 Rose Street
Franklin Park, IL 60103

STATEMENT OF PURPOSE

*   This College has been founded to gather together those physicians who wish to cooperate with families who choose to give birth in the home, the natural and traditional place for birth throughout the world and the ages. We also wish to learn from and teach each other the art of the safe supervision of homebirths.

*   Members and fellows are guided by an awareness that pregnancy, labor, and delivery are normal, physiological processes, not pathological events. We rely on these natural processes whenever feasible, reserving operative intervention of any kind or magnitude and the giving of medications for those cases where there is probability of damage to mother or baby without such intervention.

*   We take our ethic from the Hippocratic Oath and the World Medical Society Declaration at Geneva in 1948.

*   We try to foster not only the welfare of our patients, mother and baby, but that of the entire family.

*   Applications for membership are being accepted from physicians who share our philosophy and are attending homebirths.

OFFICERS

Gregory White, MD	President
Mayer Eisenstein, MD	Vice President
Herbert Ratner, MD	Secretary-Treasurer

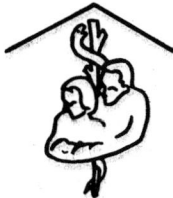

What Is NAPSAC ?

The *National Association of Parents & Professionals for Safe Alternatives in Childbirth* is dedicated to exploring, examining, implementing, and establishing Family-Centered Childbirth Programs . . . programs that meet the needs of families as well as provide the safe aspects of medical science.

Our Goals Are:

*   To promote education about the principles of Natural Childbirth.

*   To act as a forum facilitating communication and cooperation among Parents, Medical Professionals, and Childbirth Educators.

*   To encourage and aid in the implementation of Family-Centered Maternity Care in Hospitals.

*   To assist in the establishment of Maternity and Childbearing Centers.

*   To help establish Safe Homebirth Programs.

*   To provide educational opportunities to parents and to parents-to-be that will enable them to assume more personal responsibility for Pregnancy, Childbirth, Infant Care, and Child Rearing.

About Membership in NAPSAC

If you would like to receive the NAPSAC News quarterly, to be kept informed of upcoming NAPSAC programs & publications, and participate in some of the NAPSAC activities - you may become a member. Annual dues: $6.00

SEND: NAME - ADDRESS - PHONE - SPECIALTY OR MAJOR INTEREST
          With cash or check payable to NAPSAC

TO: Membership Director, NAPSAC, Box 1307, Chapel Hill, NC 27514
       until June 1, 1978, after which write to Box 267, Marble Hill,
       MO 63764

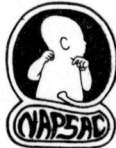

National Association of Parents & Professionals for Safe Alternatives in Childbirth

If you would like to start a NAPSAC Member Group, write to the NAPSAC Membership Director.

NAPSAC

Address until June 1, 1978:
NAPSAC, P.O. Box 1307
Chapel Hill, NC 27514
Phone (919) 732-7302

Address after June 1, 1978:
NAPSAC, P.O. Box 267
Marble Hill, MO 63764
Phone Area Code 314

INSTITUTE FOR CHILDBIRTH & FAMILY RESEARCH
a Division of NAPSAC
2522 Dana Street, Berkeley, CA 94704 (415) 849-3665

Lewis Mehl, MD ICFR Director of Research
Gail Peterson, MSSW Assistant Director of Research

The ICFR carries out the research activities of NAPSAC, Inc.,
and is a corporate division of NAPSAC. The ICFR distributes
reprints of its on going research and past publications. To
obtain information, write directly to the ICFR.

NAPSAC BOARD OF CONSULTANTS

George J. Annas, JD, MPH, *Boston, Massachusetts*
Sallee Berman, RN, CCE, AAHCC, *Culver City, California*
Victor Berman, MD, ACOG, AAHCC, *Culver City, California*
James Brew, MD, FACOG, FACS, *Washington, D.C.*
Neil Collins, JD, *Research Triangle Park, North Carolina*
James Dingfelder, MD, ACOG, *Chapel Hill, North Carolina*
Daniel Domizio, PA, *Barbuda, West Indies*
Margot Edwards, RN, MA, *Pacific Grove, California*
Janet Epstein, RN, CNM, *Bethesda, Maryland*
Doris Haire, DMS, *Hillside, New Jersey*
John Haire, JD, *Hillside, New Jersey*
Marjie Hathaway, CCET, AAHCC, *Sherman Oaks, California*
Jay Hathaway, CCET, AAHCC, *Sherman Oaks, California*
Lester Dessez Hazell, MA, *San Francisco, California*
Betty Hosford, RN, CNM, *New York City, New York*
James Little, RPT, AAHCC, *Durham, North Carolina*
Marion F. McCartney, RN, CNM, *Washington, D.C.*
Lewis Mehl, MD, ACHO, *Madison, Wisconsin*
Robert Mendelsohn, MD, ACHO, *Chicago, Illinois*
Nancy Mills, Lay Midwife, *Forestville, California*
Herbert Ratner, MD, ACHO, *Oak Park, Illinois*
Charles Taylor, MD, ACOG, *Oklahoma City, Oklahoma*
Marian Tompson, LLLI, *Franklin Park, Illinois*
Gregory White, MD, ACHO, *River Forest, Illinois*
Ruth Wilf, CNM, PHD, *Philadelphia, Pennsylvania*

Selected Abbreviations
for Titles and Organizations

AAHCC	American Academy of Husband-Coached Childbirth
ACHI	Association for Childbirth at Home, International
ACHO	American College of Home Obstetrics
ACNM	American College of Nurse-Midwives
ACOG	American College of Obstetricians & Gynecologists
ACS	American College of Surgeons
ASPO	American Society for Psychoprophylaxis in Obstetrics
BS	Bachelor of Science
CCE	Certified Childbirth Educator
CCET	Certified Childbirth Educator Trainer
CNM	Certified Nurse-Midwife
DBA	Doctor of Business Administration
DMS	Doctor of Medical Science
FACOG	Fellow, Am. College of Obstetricians & Gynecologists
FACS	Fellow, American College of Surgeons
HOME	Home Oriented Maternity Experience
ICFR	Institute for Childbirth and Family Research
ICEA	International Childbirth Education Association
JD	Doctor of Jurisprudence
LLLI	La Leche League International
LM	Lay Midwife
MA	Master of Arts
MD	Doctor of Medicine
MPH	Master of PUblic Health
MSSW	Master of Science in Social Work
NMA	National Midwives Association
PA	Physician's Associate
PHD	Doctor of Philosophy
RN	Registered Nurse
RPT	Registered Physical Therapist
SPUN	Society for the Protection of the Unborn Thru Nutrition

SELECTED RESOURCE ORGANIZATIONS

AAHCC P.O. Box 5224 Sherman Oaks, CA 91413	*Certifying and Training Agency for childbirth educators in the Bradley Method*
ACHI 1675 Monte Cristo Cerritos, CA 90701	*Instruction on homebirth for couples, with or without a birth attendant; trains teachers also.*
ACHO 2821 Rose Street Franklin Park, IL 60131	*Support, information, and training for physicians in home birth (see p. 183).*
ACNM 1000 Vermont Avenue NW Washington, DC 20005	*Certifying agency for nurse-midwives, both in home and in hospital practice.*
ASPO 1411 K Street NW Washington, DC 20005	*Certifying and Training Agency for childbirth educators in the Lamaze Method.*
HOME 511 New York Avenue Takoma Park, Wash. DC 20012	*Instruction on homebirth for couples, emphasis on medically attended birth; trains leaders.*
ICFR 2522 Dana Street Berkeley, CA 94704	*Research Division of NAPSAC, Inc. studies all aspects of birth & the family; distributes reprints.*
ICEA P.O. Box 20852 Milwaukee, WI 53220	*All aspects of childbirth education; emphasis on birth preparation and family-centered hospital care*
LLLI 9616 Minneapolis Avenue Franklin Park, IL 60131	*Support and information on breast-feeding; distributes scientific reprints; trains leaders.*
NAPSAC P.O. Box 1307 ** Chapel Hill, NC 27514	*All aspects of birth; emphasis on providing coordinated alternatives both in and out-of-hospital.*
NMA P.O. Box 163 Princeton, NJ 08540	*An association of practicing mid-wives, largely lay midwives, but some nurse midwives also.*
SPUN 17 N. Wabash, Suite 603 Chicago, IL 60602	*Education in nutrition in pregnancy; training seminars, brochures, on benefits and specifics of good diet.*

** NOTE: After June 1, 1978, NAPSAC's address will be:
P.O. Box 267, Marble Hill, MO 63764. Phone Area Code (314)

IF YOU LIKE "SAFE ALTERNATIVES IN CHILDBIRTH". .
YOU WILL ALSO LIKE "21ST CENTURY OBSTETRICS NOW!" . .

In 21st Century Obstetrics Now! the medical, psychological, sociologic,
and economic benefits of out-of-hospital birth alternatives is even more
thoroughly presented and documented, along with presentations of
establishment medicine arguing for total hospitalization of all birthing
mothers.

34 Chapters, 611 pages, over 500 cited references, original research
never before published, written for parents, yet documented for
professionals. It is the most up to date and comprehensive anthology
yet published in the field.

In the October 1977 issue of the New Age Magazine in review of both
"Safe Alternatives..." and "21st Century..." the two books were refered
to as occupying "a category all their own. . . . these books represent
the leading edge of thinking in the childbirth field. . . . scrupulously
documented . . . . the established medical community cannot dismiss
this work as the ravings of a 'lunatic fringe'. . . . also present invalua-
ble primary research. One can only hope that NAPSAC's work flourishes
and that their publications become required reading for practitioners in
the childbirth field."

Available in Quality Paperback. Price: $11 per 2-vol set or $6.50 for either
volume singly.

Order direct from NAPSAC, Box 1307, Chapel Hill, NC 27514 until June
of 1978.

After June 1, 1978, order from NAPSAC, Box 267, Marble Hill, NC 63764.

Enclose 70¢ for postage and handling (or 50 ¢ if only one of the two volumes
is ordered.

TABLE OF CONTENTS LISTED ON NEXT PAGE . . . .

21st Century Obstetrics Now!

Volume One | Volume Two

INDEX*
TO SAFE ALTERNATIVES IN CHILDBIRTH

---

* Indexed for the Third Edition by Jamy Braun, RN.

INDEX CONT'D

INDEX CONT'D

INDEX CONT'D

Pregnancy
  drugs during, 2, 17-22, 38-44, 47
    See also Analgesics &
    Analgesia and Anesthetics
    & Anesthesia.
  nutrition during, 24, 38-39, 59, 68, 75
  smoking, 55
  toxemia of, 17, 39-41
  weight during, 38-39, 59, 68, 75
Premature Infant, 32-34, 42
Prenatal Care, 8, 54-55, 104, 116-117, 131-132

R
Regionalization, 2, 15, 33
Rooming-in, 28, 155
Rupture of Membranes, 2, 16, 19, 20, 40, 44, 46-47, 76, 110

S
Separation
  of mother & baby afterbirth, 11, 19, 145-46, 159
  of mother & Siblings, 5

Sibling Participation. See Children.
Sibling Rivalry, 5
Sibling Participation. See Children.
Silver Nitrate, Eye Drops, 76, 105, 122, 132, 176
  legality of, 176
Smoking in Pregnancy, 55
Society for the Protection of the Unborn Thru Nutrition, (SPUN), 187
Stirrups, 19, 48, 59
Supine Position, 16, 44, 47-49, 59

T
Toxemia of Pregnancy, 17, 39-41

U
Ultrasound, 19

W
Weight, During Pregnancy, 38-39, 59, 68, 75. Also see Nutrition.

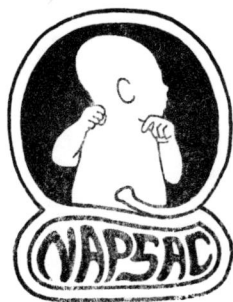

NAPSAC, INC., IS NON-PROFIT AND TAX EXEMPT.

(CONTRIBUTIONS TO NAPSAC ARE TAX DEDUCTIBLE.)